PLANNING
FOR
UNCERTAINTY

*Living Wills and
Other Advance Directives
for You and Your Family*

SECOND EDITION

DAVID JOHN DOUKAS, M.D.
WILLIAM REICHEL, M.D.

THE JOHNS HOPKINS UNIVERSITY PRESS
Baltimore

Note to the reader: This book has been written to help the reader make decisions about his or her values relating to medical care and other issues pertaining to the quality of life. This book is not meant to substitute for the advice of medical professionals or legal counsel, and neither medical nor legal decisions should be based solely on its contents.

Both editions of this book have been reviewed by legal counsel. The authors and publisher thank both attorneys for their assistance.

© 1993, 2007 The Johns Hopkins University Press
All rights reserved. Published 2007
Printed in the United States of America on acid-free paper
9 8 7 6 5 4 3 2 1

The Johns Hopkins University Press
2715 North Charles Street
Baltimore, Maryland 21218-4363
www.press.jhu.edu

Library of Congress Cataloging-in-Publication Data

Doukas, David John.
Planning for uncertainty : living wills and other advance directives for you and your family / David John Doukas, William Reichel. — 2nd ed.
p. cm. — (Johns Hopkins Press health book)
Includes index.
ISBN-13: 978-0-8018-8607-2 (hardcover : alk. paper)
ISBN-13: 978-0-8018-8608-9 (pbk. : alk. paper)
ISBN-10: 0-8018-8607-4 (hardcover : alk. paper)
ISBN-10: 0-8018-8608-2 (pbk. : alk. paper)
1. Right to die—United States. 2. Medical care—Law and legislation—United States. 3. Power of attorney—United States. 4. Patients—Legal status, laws, etc.—United States. I. Reichel, William, 1937– II. Title.
KF3827.E87D68 2007
344.7304'197—dc22
2006030212

A catalog record for this book is available from the British Library.

Contents

7

You, Your Family, and Health Care Decisions:
Choosing a Proxy   88

8

Signing Advance Directives   98

Preface

As family physicians committed to the idea that patients have a right to express their preferences in medical care, we're glad you're reading this book. Much has happened in the health care world since the first edition of *Planning for Uncertainty* was published in 1993. Relevant events that were covered widely in the media, such as the Terri Schiavo case, laid open the problem of how we need to help our loved ones discontinue treatment in the face of family disagreement and schism. As a result, more people now recognize the importance of learning about advance directives for medical care. We hope that this book will help you make decisions about your health care and inspire you to take action to ensure that your preferences are followed should you become unable to state your wishes.

Both of us have seen many instances in which a simple statement of medical care preferences or the designation of an alternate decision maker has prevented undue, unwanted medical hardship on a patient and needless sorrow for the family. And, sadly, we have also seen many cases in which the lack of such a document caused family members great anguish and caused the patient to suffer needlessly, such as in the Schiavo case in Florida. As a result, we felt compelled to revise and rewrite our book explaining advance directives and the importance of understanding values and preferences—and the importance of conveying them to family and other loved ones.

We can't overemphasize the fact that our experience tells us that you need to make such preparations *now*. No one ever knows when the time of need might arrive. Our departure from this world is a natural part of our being here. We all know that death will come at some time, but none of us knows exactly when. We wrote this book for everyone who wants to plan ahead for that time.

In the Introduction that follows we provide an overview of advance directive decision making in health care and discuss why and how to prepare an advance directive. We also discuss the law that was intended to promote advance directives, the Patient Self-Determination Act. Chapter 1 provides more information about the background and implications of this act.

In chapter 2, we describe our concept of the difference between beneficial medical care and treatment that has no benefit. In chapter 3, we explore how ethical principles may conflict when health care decisions are made. Chapter 4 explains how you might go about exploring your own values regarding when to continue—and when to refuse—medical care.

Chapter 5 discusses in detail the use of the living will and the durable power of attorney for health care. Chapter 6 takes up the subject of an innovative document called the Values History, which combines the virtues of values, the living will, and the durable power of attorney for health care. The implications of family cooperation and interference in your future medical care are discussed in chapter 7. Chapter 8 examines many issues related to advance directives and explains how to complete the advance directive forms.

In the Appendix you will find information about how to obtain copies of the durable power of attorney for health care and the living will, as well as state-specific forms for the durable power of attorney for health care, the living will, and the Values History.

Our hope is that the information in this book will allow you to make an informed decision about advance directives, so that you can confidently face future medical situations.

Acknowledgments

This book represents the experiences of two physicians and the journey they have taken in their profession. We have each had intense experience in our work in family practice, internal medicine, geriatrics, and medical ethics. We are especially grateful to our patients, whose life stories have been the single greatest educational lesson for us as physicians.

We also want to acknowledge our editor, Jacqueline Wehmueller, who agreed with us that recent national events made a second edition an essential project, so that the book might better aid people seeking help with their advance directives. We are most grateful for her contributions; this book is much enriched because she has been our editor.

Finally, we want to refer to our personal journeys through life. The events and experiences that we have each encountered have given direction to our work. Most of all we want to thank our families—our wives, Jeanne and Helen; our children, Caitlin, Alexander, and Christina Doukas, and Robert Reichel and Andrea Reichel Ruggeri—who were understanding and supportive while we wrote this book. We are grateful for their love, support, and graciousness, which allowed us to maintain our purpose and bring this work to fruition. Thank you.

PLANNING FOR UNCERTAINTY

Introduction:
What Every Person
Needs to Know

Suppose you were so ill or so badly injured that you could not speak for yourself. How would your loved ones and your doctor know what you wanted done? How can you make preparations today so they will know, if that should happen?

What is an advance directive?

An advance directive is an oral or written statement a person makes to tell health care professionals and the person's loved ones what forms of medical care the person would accept or would refuse in a specific medical circumstance; alternatively, or in addition, it names who should make such health care decisions if the person is unable to express his or her own wishes. Advance directives should be in writing, although in some situations, previous oral statements about treatment preferences will be honored. However, a written record can clearly state what the person wants, eliminating the possibility of uncertainty, confusion, or misinterpretation. Furthermore, in some states, refusal of life-sustaining treatment for incompetent adults is allowed only by a *written* directive.

Advance directives ultimately are tools, and their worth is based on how you use them. This book will discuss not only how to fill out these forms, but also how to engage your doctor and family so as to best communicate what you want. This communication can help insure that those persons will be well prepared to speak on your behalf someday if you cannot speak for yourself. These discussions should address a wide variety of issues and should happen, more than once, for advance care planning must be an ongoing process of in-depth discussions and reviews between you and those whom you trust.

Advance directives can be specific, addressing particular medical therapies that you wish to have or to refuse. Alternatively, advance directives can be broad, providing a blanket refusal of life-sustaining medical therapy in cases of terminal illness or irreversible coma (as in a living will). You can appoint a decision maker who will have legal power to speak for you if you are incapacitated but you still need to discuss with your loved ones what you deem appropriate versus inappropriate medical treatment in your future and how you want your family to make decisions for you.

What has generated so much recent attention about advance directives in the media and among the public?

This recent attention occurred in the wake of the famous case in Florida in 2005 regarding a young woman named Terri Schiavo.

What happened to Terri Schiavo?

A dispute between Ms. Schiavo's husband and her parents, the Schindlers, produced what many see as the most important end-of-life case since those of Karen Quinlan in the 1970s and Nancy

Cruzan in the 1980s. In February 1990, at 27 years old, Theresa (Terri) Marie Schiavo suffered a cardiac arrest (heart attack), which then caused anoxia (insufficient oxygen in her blood), resulting in severe brain damage. At the time of her cardiac arrest, Terri Schiavo had no living will, advance directive, or other written evidence of her wishes. She remained in a persistent vegetative state (PVS) for fifteen years, maintained on artificial nutrition and hydration.

Her husband, Michael, asked the court to make surrogate decisions for the discontinuation of Terri's feeding tube, which provided nutrition and hydration. The court repeatedly made this decision, based on Terri's prior oral statements to Michael and others. Terri's parents opposed the removal, based on their desire to help keep Terri alive and a belief that she was not in a persistent vegetative state and would somehow be rehabilitated with therapy.

In multiple rulings, the courts decided to withdraw the feeding tube. Unfortunately, the case became highly politicized when the Florida House of Representatives and Senate passed a bill, in 2003, dubbed "Terri's Law," which allowed Governor Jeb Bush to issue a "one time stay in certain cases." Governor Bush then issued an executive order directing reinsertion of the feeding tube and appointing a guardian ad litem for Terri Schiavo. However, Florida's Supreme Court ruled that the state's executive and legislative branches' attempts to subvert Michael's request to stop the tube feeding were improper, and that Michael Schiavo could indeed serve as Terri's proxy in this request.

How was this case resolved?

Despite repeated appeals to the U.S. Supreme Court (which declined review of the case) and attempts by the U.S. Congress to impede the discontinuation of the treatment, Michael Schiavo's request to withdraw the feeding tube was allowed. Terri Schiavo died March 31, 2005, at age 41, in a hospice in Pinellas Park,

Florida, thirteen days after the feeding tube was removed from her stomach. The autopsy on Terri Schiavo demonstrated that at her death her brain weighed 615 grams—half that of a normal adult brain. The medical examiner concluded that the condition of her brain prevented any chance of treatment or rehabilitation.

What are the repercussions of this case?

There was much public misunderstanding regarding the issues in the Terri Schiavo case. Public and political pressure was applied for lawmakers to intervene in this case. Unfortunately, interventions were based on these pressures rather than on a careful analysis of the medical facts at hand and a clearly expressed set of witnessed instructions by a person prior to lapsing into incapacity.

The biggest lesson from the Schiavo case (as well as the Quinlan and Cruzan cases, discussed later in this book) is that advance directives, when coupled with sound lines of communication with family members who can represent the patients when they cannot speak for themselves, can help prevent the unleashing of a tornado of forces. The hope is that the Terri Schiavo tragedy will spark far more conversation in people's homes about advance directive planning and reduce the possibility of family strife concerning who best represents a person's wishes.

The family is the place where we can express personal views about values, wishes, and preferences in general, but especially about death and dying. Family members are the people most familiar with our personal and religious values. In choosing family members who can be trusted, we must have conversations to make sure that the people chosen are well informed about our wishes and strong-willed enough to defend those wishes in the face of opposition from others.

How can I help prevent a dispute like the one in the Schiavo/ Schindler family from taking place someday in my own family?

In this book, we will explain how living wills and durable powers of attorney for health care can offer helpful starting points for conversations on advance care planning that are necessary for all adults. These documents are only tools, though, and they *must* be fleshed out in the fuller context of the values and preferences one has about one's future health care. In addition, these wishes must then be conveyed to one's loved ones to help make sure these wishes are carried out. The inclusion of families in the decision-making process can provide the greatest enhancement of the patient's autonomy and is the best way to avoid the woeful disputes seen in the Schiavo case.

When we express a clear and convincing preference not to have life prolonged artificially with a medical therapy (including artificial fluids and nutrition), then we have the right to have that therapy discontinued. Contrariwise, we also have a right to request those therapies that we want to have used in our care, and, if they are deemed medically appropriate, we should be able to feel sure that they will be provided. In sum, we each have the right to decide what therapies will be imposed upon our bodies and the right to accept or reject them prospectively, for the future, even if lack of a therapy may cause us to die. Importantly, no doctor or family should be allowed to overturn or refuse to accept these stated preferences in the future. At the same time, it is important to note that a doctor is not required to do things that are contrary to his or her own professional values and beliefs; this does not mean that your wishes cannot be carried out but that another doctor or health care institution may need to be found to accomplish them.

Why is an advance directive important to me?

An advance directive is needed by every adult who is competent and able to make decisions about his or her future health care. First, it is easier to make decisions when you are healthy and are able to think more objectively about these topics. While some people may find thinking about these topics distressing, we know from experience that it's better to put some thought into these matters when you're well than to wait until you become sick. Making decisions about medical care is far more likely to be difficult for a sick person. And sometimes people are too sick to be able to make these decisions at all.

Second, if you *don't* make an advance directive and later you become unable to speak for yourself, your doctor and your family may have difficulty making decisions about your care. When faced with the option that other people may have to make decisions about their care some day, most people prefer to make their own medical decisions, based on their own preferences, which can be carried out later should they become ill. Advance directives allow people to make their own choices about health care *in advance,* so that their preferences will be known when they are too sick to voice their wishes.

Third, some forms of advance directives spare the family the daunting task of making decisions for a family member who is unable to communicate. An advance directive lifts this burden from the family. An advance directive gives the family and medical team a way to use your own values and preferences, rather than making some kind of best guess about what you would want or trying to judge based on your values. The benefit of your own forward thinking becomes very clear. Of course, it is wise to pick a surrogate decision maker or proxy from among your family or friends, someone who understands your preferences, values, and beliefs. This person becomes your advocate, the one who will work with your health care team in the future if you cannot speak for yourself. Importantly, this designation can avoid the problems that arise if some family members hold values different from yours. When you select a proxy who will carry out your preferences, then you can be far more confident that family members who do not share your values will not attempt to overrule your wishes.

Why do I need to think about this now?

Even if you are in good health, you should think about medical advance directive decision making now. Procrastination is a common human failing: we put off preparing our taxes and making out our will for the disposition of our financial estate. As physicians, we have seen the unfortunate results of procrastinating about advance directives, and we must say that the results can be devastating.

Creating advance directives will prompt you to make decisions about what kinds of health care you want in the future. You can always change your mind and alter or revoke an advance directive later. If you think about this *now*, though, and you make a decision about it *now*, and you document your decision *now*, that decision will more likely be respected and be acted upon later by your health care team. If your values, preferences, or choice of a proxy changes, you are always able to change your advance directive. However, if you do not have an advance directive at all, your wishes regarding your care may be unclear to your doctor and family.

If an advance directive is so important, why doesn't everyone have one?

Despite the importance of advance directives for health care, only a small proportion of adults (fewer than 1 in 5) have executed one.

Most people haven't considered executing an advance directive because they haven't thought (or don't wish to think) about prolonged incapacity or the end of their life. It is much easier for us to think about our present needs and circumstances than it is to think about what prolonged incapacity or the end of our own life will be like, so we put off executing advance directives. Many people haven't signed an advance directive because they don't know enough about it or don't know how to get one. People may not learn about advance directives until they are completing their estate planning. While preparing a will or living trust, an attorney may provide a durable power of attorney, a living will, and a durable power of attorney for health care. Some people delay making an advance directive because they believe that they need to pay a lawyer to help them, but neither the living will nor the durable power of attorney for health care requires the involvement of an attorney. While most people find advance directives intuitively to be a good idea, the factors of procrastination and lack of understanding probably explain why so many people have not filled out an advance directive.

Another factor limiting advance directive use is that some clinicians do not place a high priority on advance health care planning. Some clinicians simply are not well informed on this subject; some may be so focused on the present clinical picture that they are not thinking of stages in which an advance directive may help the patient. Physicians often do not discuss do-not-resuscitate (DNR) orders or end-of-life issues with patients. Time constraints are influential factors today in clinical practice. In corporate medicine, demands on productivity may be the determining factor governing the physician's use of time.

Finally, many people do not understand the purpose of advance directives or living wills. A patient may think that signing a living will precludes provision of life-saving techniques in all circumstances, even a nonterminal episode, such as a first heart attack. (It does not.) A patient may not understand that advance directives and living wills are focused on the patient who is terminally ill or permanently unable to make decisions. (When you do have capacity, your say is the final say.)

This book not only will explain advance directives as helpful tools but also will relate how easy it is to obtain an advance directive and fill it out. You can get an advance directive through the web links provided in our Appendix or from your family doctor, local health department, state representative, or hospital admissions office. Private organizations such as the National Hospice and Palliative Care Organization and AARP (formerly the American Association for Retired Persons) (see the Appendix) can also provide you with one.

More older people than younger people have executed an advance directive, and people are more likely to do so as they get older. Should people wait, then, until they are older to sign an advance directive? No, we believe now is the best time. There's no way to predict when a serious accident or illness might occur, so it is prudent to make such plans now. Remember that the Karen Ann Quinlan, Nancy Cruzan, and, most recently, Terri Schiavo, cases all involved people who were in only their third decade of life. When these young women lapsed into a persistent vegetative state, their loved ones were forced to make difficult decisions about their care. The lack of an advance directive made these decisions much more painful as well as legally challenging. One sign of hope in our effort to bring about change in the number of people preparing living wills is that heightened public discussion of the Schiavo case caused an enormous surge in requests for advance directives.

What role can my physicians play in preparing an advance directive?

We believe that you should review your values and preferences with your personal physician and your loved ones before signing an advance directive (see chapter 5). The ideal is for everyone to have a personal physician and to hold conversations with that physician; we realize that many people do not enjoy continuity of care with a personal physician. A discussion with your physician will give you information and insight into the consequences of the many decisions that can be made about medical care. By discussing these matters with your personal doctor, you will have a much better understanding of what you are consenting to or refusing, and why. Signing an advance directive after careful thought and informed discussion is obviously preferable to signing with little reflection or understanding. Also, as a result of these discussions, your personal physician will have a much better understanding of your motivations and feelings.

What is a living will?

A living will is a written declaration allowing a person to direct that life-sustaining medical therapies be withdrawn or withheld if the person is terminally ill and no longer able to make decisions. Living wills are currently recognized by statute in nearly every state. In many states, living wills also apply to persons in a persistent vegetative state. (The terms *terminal illness* and *persistent vegetative state* are discussed in chapter 5.) A "generic" living will can be helpful in those states where the living will has not yet been recognized by statute (see the Appendix). A living will can tell your doctor and your family your preferences regarding life-sustaining therapies, so they have a basis upon which to act if you can no longer speak for yourself.

A living will, therefore, is a type of written advance directive. It allows you to put in writing your wish not to have life-sustaining medical therapies begun or continued if you are dying from a terminal illness and are unable to communicate. It does *not* allow you to demand treatment that would not benefit you.

What is a durable power of attorney?

The durable power of attorney gives someone you designate the legal authority to act or make decisions on your behalf. The *durable* aspect of this document is important. A (simple) power of attorney becomes void when the person who wrote it becomes incapacitated. That is, a *power of attorney* recognizes the authority of one person to act or make decisions only for another *competent* person. A *durable power of attorney* recognizes the authority of one person to act or make decisions for an *incompetent* person. This authority can be used temporarily in cases of accidents or time-limited illness, or in a long-term sense in cases of protracted, irreversible incapacity. To be *durable,* the power of attorney must include a provision similar to one of the following:

1. "This power of attorney shall not be affected by my incapacity"; or
2. "This power of attorney will take effect upon my incapacity."

The durable power of attorney is recognized in every state and the District of Columbia. In addition, some states have laws more specifically addressing durable powers of attorney for health care.

What is a durable power of attorney for health care?

A durable power of attorney for health care is a document delegating authority to another person to make decisions *specifically about health care*. It allows you to transfer your authority to whomever you choose. That person will decide which medical therapies to accept and which to refuse if you are unable to speak for yourself. The document also allows you to state your preferences regarding future medical care, so that if someday you are unable to communicate, the person speaking for you has instructions from you about what you want done and not done.

A durable power of attorney for health care is different from other durable powers of attorney in that it specifically addresses *only* health care issues. It does *not* give anyone authority to manage the person's estate or to make financial decisions. It is our understanding that every state that recognizes the durable power of attorney recognizes the durable power of attorney for health care. (Note that some states require that the durable power of attorney for business matters be a separate document from the durable power of attorney for health care.)

What is a proxy?

A proxy, also known as a *health care surrogate,* is the person selected to serve as an agent for the patient under a durable power of attorney for health care. The proxy has the power to make medical decisions for the patient when the patient is unable to do so. (In some states, the law allows someone to appoint a proxy to make decisions for the person while he or she is still competent.) The proxy uses his or her understanding of the patient's values and preferences regarding various medical therapies to make decisions about treatment. This understanding is based on previous conversations and written advance directives. The decisions made by the proxy should reflect the decisions the patient would make, given the medical circumstances under consideration, if he or she were able to. The proxy must, of course, also follow any written instructions provided by the patient in the durable power of attorney for health care, or in any other document.

If I sign an advance directive, how long will it remain in effect?

Any advance directive you sign when competent will remain in effect unless and until you revoke it. *Only you can revoke your own advance directive*. You can revoke it by completely destroying your current advance directive and, optimally, all existing copies. You can change the directive by crossing out parts or altering them before witnesses, or you can sign and date a new advance directive, which will make it clear that it replaces any others you have signed in the past. You can do this whenever you wish. In many states, revocation is allowed even if you are without mental capacity, so treatment requests from a nonlucid patient must be honored. Otherwise, the only way an advance directive can be countermanded is if you have conversations with other persons and these conversations are witnessed, and your new preferences are stated while you are lucid. In short, you can change your mind, but someone else cannot change your stated preferences for you. This aspect of using an advance directive is very important, as it expects a level of thoughtfulness about your future wishes, your attention to document these wishes, and the need to review these wishes over time and if your health should change. As no form can ever be perfect, talking with your loved ones about what you want and do not want may still be the best safeguard of your right to decide your future health care.

Where should the advance directive be kept?

Of course, it is critical that the advance directive be available when needed. It should be kept in a place that is readily accessible, so that your loved ones will be able to get it when it is needed. Make copies for your loved ones, for anyone designated in the advance directive, and for your doctor. The advance directive must not be locked away in the same vault or safe deposit box as your will or living trust. Make extra copies; advance directives may be misplaced or they may disappear during transfer of patients from one health care facility to another.

Is my advance directive legally valid everywhere?

Format and verbal preferences in advance directives vary from state to state, so an advance directive from one state could be challenged in other states. However, most states agree that valid advance directives drawn up in one jurisdiction will be useable in another jurisdiction.

1

WHAT THE PATIENT
SELF-DETERMINATION ACT
MEANS TO YOU

Suppose you were hospitalized for an unexpected illness. How does the hospital help you let your doctor and your loved ones know what you want done even if you cannot speak?

What is the Patient Self-Determination Act?

Passed by the U.S. Congress late in 1990, the Patient Self-Determination Act (PSDA) is a federal law that took effect on December 1, 1991. It requires all hospitals, nursing homes, home health agencies, hospices, and health maintenance organizations that receive Medicare or Medicaid funds to provide patients with a written statement of their rights, under that state's laws, to accept or refuse treatment and to prepare advance directives for health care. The Patient Self-Determination Act also requires these institutions to ask patients if they have signed an advance directive, and it prohibits discrimination against patients on the basis of whether or not they have signed an advance directive. In some facilities, living will and durable power of attorney forms may be available to patients, and signed advance directives may be photocopied and placed in the medical record. The medical system of the Department of Veterans Affairs has its own version of the PSDA's requirements. If you have been hospitalized or have entered a home care situation or nursing home or have joined a health maintenance organization (HMO) since the PSDA was enacted, you should have been asked about advance directives upon entry.

The Patient Self-Determination Act helped achieve the passage of advance directive legislation in all states. The act was also intended to educate physicians, nurses, health care administrators, and consumers about advance directives. Congress hoped that the law would result in increased citizen awareness of the living will and the durable power of attorney for health care, but here the PSDA fell short of its goal.

Part of the stimulus for the introduction of this legislation was the unfortunate case of Nancy Cruzan in 1990 and public debate about the case. Like the recent Terri Schiavo case, this prominent case dealt with a very difficult situation involving a request to withdraw a feeding tube from a young woman who was in a persistent vegetative state (this case is discussed in chapter 8).

What is the Patient Self-Determination Act supposed to do?

The Patient Self-Determination Act is intended to ensure that all patients are made aware of their rights concerning health care and advance directive decisions at the time of admission to hospitals and other health care settings. The act affords patients an opportunity, if they wish, to learn about and prepare an advance directive before they become incompetent or unable to do so. Of course, when one is being admitted to the hospital is not a conducive time to discuss advance directives, given the anxiety, stress, and pain that the patient may have then and the additional anxiety that thinking about incapacitation and end-of-life issues may cause.

How does the Patient Self-Determination Act work?

According to the Patient Self-Determination Act, all patients being admitted to a health care institution that receives Medicare or Medicaid funds will be given written information about their legal rights regarding advance directives and the institution's policies for honoring those rights. This process is to take place at the time of admission, unless the patient's condition makes it impracticable. Materials on the institution's advance directives policy must also be provided. In addition, the patient (or the patient's legal representative) must be asked during the admissions process whether he or she already has signed an advance directive. The institution's counsel or administration may provide, if the patient requests them, specific materials on living wills and durable powers of attorney.

If it is not an emergency when the patient is admitted to the hospital, the admissions clerk (or possibly a social worker or nurse) may give the patient a written statement describing the health care institution's obligations to honor patients' health care requests, including advance directives. We believe it is unfortunate that there is no mandate that such discussions be initiated by the patient's primary care physician.

If the patient has signed a living will or durable power of attorney, this fact must be entered into the patient's medical record. At this point, hospitals typically enter copies of advance directives into the patient's medical record if the patient has signed one—in fact, most states' advance directive laws *require* that a copy of the signed advance directive be placed in the patient's record. If the patient has not signed an advance directive, he or she may be given materials to consider regarding signing an advance directive. Such information is usually available to the patient from the admissions or patient services office in the hospital.

In some circumstances, for example, when a patient enters the hospital in an emergency and is unconscious, the first concern is to provide medical care. In such an event, a designated person on the hospital's staff will provide the hospital's advance directive policy materials to the patient's proxy or family member (if they have accompanied the patient) and ask if the patient has signed an advance directive. If the patient has signed an advance directive, a copy of the advance directive will be placed in the patient's medical record as soon as it can be brought to the hospital.

In reality, this could become (and often is) an automatic and trivialized process. When a patient is admitted to the hospital, the admissions clerk may ask whether he or she has a living will or durable power of attorney. If the clerk merely accepts an affirmative response then enters this information into the record, gives the patient a policy sheet on advance directives, and moves on, certain important issues will not have been addressed. The location of the advance directive (accessibility is crucial) and the naming of an agent through a durable power of attorney (location and willingness of the agent are important) are matters that could be overlooked. Merely asking if you have an advance directive is not enough. The lesson here is: If you have an advance directive, bring a copy of it with you when you are electively hospitalized, and if you are admitted on an emergency basis, have someone bring the document as soon as they can.

After the admissions process, if interactions with health professionals do not include mention or discussion of advance directives, the patient may not have an adequate opportunity to convey the intent of his or her directive. We believe that there should be not only basic communication with patients about their consent to or refusal of medical treatments but also discussion of the meaning of these decisions.

Further, under the Patient Self-Determination Act, these health care institutions have an obligation to train their staff and educate the public concerning the options of advance directive use. Unfortunately, as in certain other pieces of legislation that Congress has passed, no money was allocated to cover the expense of these educational efforts or the distribution of advance directives to patients. Indeed, since no special training was mandated for members of the health care staff providing the patient with information, quality control for the process of informing patients has been a concern. Nevertheless, hospitals and other health agencies appear to be doing their best to carry out the PSDA mandate, despite the additional time and money required.

A final provision of the law mandates that each state develop or approve the written materials on advance directives that will be given to patients, and that the federal government develop similar materials for distribution to health professionals and beneficiaries of Social Security, while at the same time developing a national educational effort on advance directives for the general population.

Which staff member is responsible for asking the patient about advance directives?

The PSDA leaves this up to the facility. This is one of the areas of weakness of the law. We have already pointed out that the law does not mandate that physicians ask about and discuss advance directives with the patient and that this role often is carried out by the admissions clerk (and in some cases by social workers or nurses). We believe that the law is relying on inpatient or institutional settings to carry out a function that should take place over a period of time in the outpatient or office setting. With the exception of the requirement of the law that applies to health maintenance organizations, the law does not encourage people to prepare an advance directive before hospitalization or nursing home placement becomes necessary. Finally, as mentioned above, at the time the person reaches the hospital or long-term facility, he or she may not be competent to discuss treatment preferences, choices, or values. These are problems that must be addressed by patients and their doctors in order to improve upon the original intent of the Patient Self-Determination Act.

What is a Medicare- or Medicaid-receiving health care institution?

Most hospitals, nursing homes, hospices, home health agencies, and health maintenance organizations receive payments from Medicare or Medicaid. If they do, they are subject to the requirements of the Patient Self-Determination Act.

What happens if the act is not followed?

If the hospitals or health agencies do not follow the provisions of the Patient Self-Determination Act, they risk losing eligibility to receive Medicare and Medicaid payments. The Congress believes that this risk provides sufficient motivation for them to comply with the act, and so far that seems to hold true in most cases.

Will I only be asked about advance directives if I'm being admitted to a health care facility or being enrolled in a health maintenance organization?

At this time under the Patient Self-Determination Act, it is when you are being admitted to a hospital, nursing home, home health agency, or hospice, or being enrolled in a health maintenance organization that you must be asked about your advance directives. However, you may come across materials on this subject in doctors' offices, clinics, and other outpatient settings, as well. Doctors should discuss advance directives with their patients during routine office visits, and some do.

Who else should talk with me about advance directives?

Discussions prompted by the Patient Self-Determination Act at Medicare- and Medicaid-funded facilities are not the only discussions you ought to have about advance directive options. It's a good idea to sit down with your doctor (if you have one) to discuss the advance directives that are recognized in your state. Write down what you would like to have done in the future if you are ever terminally ill or are unable to express your wishes about medical treatment. You may also be asked about advance directives when you are planning your financial estate with your attorney.

In any case, now is the appropriate time to consider filling out an advance directive, because your current interest in this topic suggests that you appreciate the wisdom of signing one, and your understanding of this subject will have been enhanced by reading this book. The more information on advance directives you have, the more informed your choices will be when you sign one. That is why we describe the types of advance directives in detail in the upcoming chapters.

Whether the Patient Self-Determination Act will someday be extended to outpatient clinics and private doctors' offices is presently unknown. In our view, such an approach would clearly be beneficial to all patients.

Is this just more admissions paperwork?

We hope not, but the potential exists. If patients are given only the minimum of required information, that information may be reduced to a few written pages that could easily be shuffled into the rest of the admissions paperwork (the consent forms and insurance information, for example).

Nothing could be more counter to the spirit of the Patient Self-Determination Act than burying the patient under an avalanche of paper into which the material on advance directives is shuffled, perhaps never to be seen by the patient. To make sure this doesn't happen to you, you can learn about advance directives and fill them out now, before you have to go to a hospital or nursing home, and take the signed directives with you if you need admission.

How does this law help me?

If advance directive materials make you search inside yourself to decide what your wishes are and how you would like certain medical care decisions carried out, then the Patient Self-Determination Act would appear to be helping you. If you don't understand the materials, you can always speak to a doctor, nurse, or someone else who can explain the document and help you express your wishes. Don't hesitate to ask for assistance.

Have objections to the Patient Self-Determination Act been raised?

Yes, there have been several points of contention. Some people have argued that advance directives are already widely available. Yet, the rate of signing has been quite low, even after passage of the Patient Self-Determination Act. Others have argued that it is the patient's responsibility, or that it is too uncomfortable for doctors to speak to patients about death and advance directives, or that the requirements of the PSDA might upset the patient who is being admitted to the hospital or long-term facility. However, we believe that the right of the patient to give an informed consent (discussed in chapter 3) is reason enough to conform to the act.

Some people contend that this act should only apply to the elderly and debilitated. But many people become terminally ill or have serious accidents that leave them persistently vegetative. Also, although health care institutions are prohibited under the

PSDA from requiring an advance directive, some people argue that the act could indirectly coerce patients to sign advance directives, so that the health care institution will save the costs of end-of-life care. Such behavior by institutions has not been seen. This concern is important, however, for it illustrates today's collision between cost-containment in medicine and the freedom of the patient to make a decision. The ability of any institution to intrude into an individual's ability to consent to a therapy is ethically unacceptable to us, whether or not such intrusion profits a hospital or society as a whole.

If these objections aren't convincing, do you see any problems with this law?

In our view, the Patient Self-Determination Act *does* have shortcomings. As discussed above, for example, the act does not require that physicians talk to patients; rather, the exchange of information can occur at the admissions desk, along with the rest of the paperwork given to the patient at this time. This lack of contact between physician and patient undermines efforts toward educating patients about advance directives and gaining their consent.

Also, outpatient medical facilities and clinics (except health maintenance organizations, hospices, and home health agencies) are not affected by the act. Yet, patients admitted to the hospital are not optimal candidates for advance directive decision making, for they may be in pain, they may be fearful, or they may not be able to respond. We believe strongly that efforts to educate patients about advance directives should also be a priority in the outpatient health care setting. Doctors owe it to all their adult patients to routinely discuss personal choices about health care, including the choice of refusing treatment in the event of terminal illness or incompetence, so that patients have an opportunity to voice their preferences.

What improvements in the PSDA might be in the offing?

The Patient Self-Determination Act could be improved in a variety of ways that might broaden its scope. It could recommend that discussions between physicians and patients be offered in all medical offices, clinics, and health care institutions. Money could be allocated to fund public service programs and programs for medical staff to educate them about the use of advance directives. Attorneys and health insurance companies could more actively encourage the use of advance directives among their clients. All of these proposals might be given greater attention if the public demands it of legislators, attorneys, and insurance companies.

2

WHEN IS TREATMENT BENEFICIAL AND WHEN IS IT NOT BENEFICIAL?

Suppose you became so ill that no treatment would heal you or stop your suffering. How would your loved ones and your doctor know what treatments you would consider to be not beneficial?

What are life-sustaining therapies?

Life-sustaining therapies are medical treatments that prolong a person's life; they will keep you alive. They may not return you to your previous state of health. There are many kinds of treatment that are life sustaining, including breathing machines (respirators or ventilators), feeding tubes (inserted through your nose or abdomen into your stomach), and intravenous hydration and medication (fluids given through a vein). These therapies are discussed in detail in chapter 6. In our view, life-sustaining therapy may be appropriate at certain times and not appropriate at others. We discuss below the difference between these two times.

What is heroic therapy?

Although the term *heroic therapy* has fallen into disfavor, many of our patients and colleagues, as well as the media, continue to use it. It is rooted in an historical concept of patient heroism in fighting disease, and in the past was applied to life-sustaining therapy. In current usage it refers to extraordinary procedures that can endanger a patient's life as well as possibly save it. The more precise term *life-sustaining treatment* is far preferable to the dated term *heroic therapy,* as there are times when a treatment will not benefit or meaningfully sustain the life of the patient.

What are nutrition and hydration?

Nutrition, as a medical term, refers to a broad range of means of providing nutrients (food or specially prepared liquid formulas) to a patient. These methods include self-provided nutrition (feeding oneself by mouth); oral nutrition provided by someone else (spoon-feeding); artificial nutrition provided by inserting a tube through the nose down to the stomach or the small intestine (a nasogastric tube), so that liquefied food can be delivered; artificial nutrition provided by surgically inserting a tube into the stomach or into the small intestine (a gastrostomy tube), so that liquid nutrition can be supplied; and artificial nutrition provided by putting a tube into a vein, so that simple nutrients in a liquid form can be delivered directly into the bloodstream. Nutrition is termed artificial when it is provided by tubes requiring medical and technical intervention to insert them into the body. *Hydration* is defined as providing water, often supplemented with chemicals, to maintain a proper chemical balance in the bloodstream.

The use of nutrition and hydration are often considered together in medical decisions because they are often administered together. They provide the necessary sustenance while the patient is unable to swallow food, and they help the patient avoid malnutrition and chemical imbalances.

Discontinuation of nutrition and hydration will inevitably lead to death. Some people feel uncomfortable about stopping nutrition and hydration because they believe that doing so is depriving the patient of basic social and nutritional requirements and that doing so will inflict suffering. (Indeed, some living will statutes prohibit the withholding or withdrawal of artificial nutrition and hydration unless there is an explicitly stated preference that they be withheld or discontinued.) On the other hand, many physicians and patients believe that nutrition and hydration are like other medical therapies that patients are entitled to refuse. This is the position taken by virtually all the courts that have considered the question, as well as by the American Medical Association.

One point needs to be made about the concern over causing pain: stopping nutrition and hydration is usually considered when the person is near the end of life or has markedly diminished brain function. The discontinuation of such therapy usually is combined with the administration of pain-relieving medications, to ensure that the person feels no discomfort.

For example, consider the case of a woman with terminal cancer who has written a living will specifically requesting the discontinuation of nutrition and hydration if she becomes terminally ill and is no longer able to communicate. The actual withdrawal (that is, the removal of the various tubes from her body) may take but an instant, yet the process of her dying may take several days. During this process, efforts would be made to ensure that she does not feel discomfort from dehydration. Comfort care measures would be taken—her mouth would be moistened and she would be kept clean. Medicines would still be administered to alleviate her pain. If she became unconscious, the probability that she would perceive pain is even more remote, but minimizing the chance of her experiencing pain would help her and reassure her family. Remember that we are discussing the discontinuation of treatment. We never stop *caring for* patients.

Is stopping life-sustaining treatment like suicide or killing?

It is our belief that stopping life-sustaining treatment when a patient is terminally ill or persistently vegetative is not like suicide or active killing, because the withdrawal or withholding of therapy is not the cause of the person's death. (This is also the position taken by most courts and state statutes.) Rather, the therapy is merely prolonging the person's life while the disease or condition is killing the patient.

Some people think that if they forgo the use of a ventilator or a feeding tube, they will be committing suicide, or that if they request the cessation of such care for someone else, they will be engaging in a form of murder. This kind of thinking is both ethically and legally not correct. Forgoing therapy allows the disease to progress as it would without medical intervention. As most courts and state legislatures have stated, forgoing therapy for a terminally ill person allows life to end more naturally by letting the disease run its course.

Is stopping a therapy the same as never starting it?

Patients and their families often ask this question. The distinction between withholding or not starting a therapy and stopping a therapy is artificial. The law makes no such distinction. The two options need to be viewed in the same light, for three reasons.

First, if a patient could never stop a therapy once started, he or she could never *try* a therapy. Placing such a restriction—that therapy must be continued, once started—on the use of life-sustaining treatment is fallacious, because the initiation of a treatment would require its being continued indefinitely.

Second, people have a right to refuse medical therapies, and this applies to therapies already begun as well as to those yet to be initiated. Because a treatment is life sustaining does not mean that a person cannot refuse that therapy or stop its use.

Finally, the notion that stopping a therapy is a form of suicide or killing is also incorrect, for the reasons stated above. Therefore, if the patient (or his or her proxy) wishes to stop a therapy, he or she ought to be allowed to do so. It is the illness that kills, not the person who stops the therapy.

What are "benefits" and "burdens"?

The terms *benefits* and *burdens* are often used when discussing whether or not a medical therapy should be started or discontinued. When a person considers whether a therapy is worth using, he or she first determines if the benefits gained by accepting that therapy outweigh the burdens endured by accepting that therapy.

How does a patient weigh benefits and burdens?

Benefits and burdens can't simply be quantified and then weighed against each other. The respective weight assigned to a harm and a benefit will be influenced by many factors, such as the values of the patient, the memories the patient has of his or her own past illnesses and those of family and friends, and the patient's attitude toward the illness.

Consider the person who has a nasogastric tube (a tube passed through the nose down the esophagus to the stomach or small intestine for administration of liquid nutrition and hydration). That tube may be uncomfortable, and yet it may be the only means by which the person can stay alive. The benefit is that the person is sustained nutritionally with that tube. It is not uncommon, however, for a person who is being fed through such a tube to develop repeated pneumonias. These lung infections occur because the liquid food, after being delivered to the stomach through the tube, can back up into the esophagus (which connects the mouth to the stomach) to the windpipe, and from there into the lungs.

A person who has had repeated pneumonias from the food administered in this way may experience these infections as a burden resulting from the tube. If the person is terminally ill, the nutritional benefit of keeping the tube in place may not be worth the burden of repeated pneumonia. People who have seen a friend or family member go through a similar experience may respond to such memories by indicating that they believe the burden outweighs the potential benefit of this treatment.

What's involved in weighing benefits and burdens?

Weighing benefits and burdens is a difficult thing to do because it must be done on a case-by-case basis. Diseases differ, and so does the severity of illnesses. Not everyone values or weighs benefits and burdens in the same way. For these reasons, benefits and burdens must be weighed on an individualized basis.

Sometimes the weighing of benefits and burdens takes place between the physician and the patient's family, after the patient can no longer speak. That's one reason it's a good idea to discuss with your family and your physician what treatments you consider burdensome—so that other people will understand how you define an unbearable burden. (Such discussions may take place over an extended time.) Having conversations with family members helps convey this information for use in the future, enhancing the communication and easing any potential anxiety about what to do in the future.

How does my notion of benefit versus burden affect my preferences?

Your definition of beneficial treatment and your definition of burdensome treatment will determine to some degree what you need to discuss with your family and with your physician. You may have strong feelings about which types of medical illness (and their degree of severity) should be treated and which types (and severity) should not be treated by any form of medical treatment. It is best to document your beliefs in a clear-cut way in an advance directive.

The decisions you make need to be well informed, and you also need to have some understanding of the implications of medical scenarios that can occur in your future. For this reason, you need to know something about the outcomes of different types of disease. Yet, you can't be expected to predict the future—you can only speculate on the reasonable outcomes of your current health status, with the risk factors you know about, including family disease history and your own use of tobacco, drugs, and alcohol. People with lung disease who continue to smoke cigarettes, for example, may already have decided how they feel about being placed on a ventilator (breathing machine) if their lungs suddenly stopped working.

What is nonbeneficial treatment?

Nonbeneficial treatment is any treatment for which there is no medical evidence supporting its use, no physiologic reason it will benefit the patient, and no palliative merit. Palliative therapies are those designed to keep the patient comfortable. A medical treatment may be considered nonbeneficial to start or nonbeneficial to continue. Thus, some treatments may be nonbeneficial even if they are not burdensome (because they don't improve the patient's condition). A treatment is considered nonbeneficial if it would have no demonstrable medical benefit for *this* patient. For someone who is in the last stages of a terminal illness, curative treatments would be considered without benefit. Often, at this point of illness, palliative care (comfort care) can be most valuable.

Is the doctor obliged to discuss nonbeneficial treatment with a patient?

Some doctors would say no. In their view, because the treatment isn't beneficial, there is no requirement to bring it up. Other doctors say yes. Because the patient may have expectations of receiving certain treatments as his or her life is ending, these doctors reason (and we agree), the patient should be informed that these treatments would not help.

More than likely, your doctor will be forthright in telling you if some treatment may be nonbeneficial for you in your circumstances. On the other hand, your doctor may not believe that it is ever necessary to offer or discuss nonbeneficial treatments. If you sense that this is the case, you may want to have a serious talk with the doctor, to inform him or her of your desire to be kept informed of your health status and options, even if treatments are no longer of benefit. If your doctor is honest with you about your condition, you can prepare yourself for the time you have remaining, knowing that medical treatments will no longer be beneficial.

Physicians should not offer a treatment if it has no benefit, but we believe they should at least explain why such treatment would not help the patient. In any event, physicians are not required to *provide* nonbeneficial treatment. We believe that if there is no benefit to a treatment, the patient has no right to demand that the doctor provide it. A question remains, though:

Is benefit the same for everyone?

No, it is not. In our view, the notion of benefit must be related to the age and overall medical condition of the patient. The healthier the patient, the higher the expectation of recovery; hence, the higher the likelihood that medical treatments will be beneficial. (We further discuss the impact of age and illness on medical decision making in chapter 8.) Medical therapies that are appropriate for a strong young adult who contracts a reversible illness are much more likely to succeed than the same therapies for the same illness but administered to an elderly patient with multiple medical problems, chronic disease, or terminal illness. The concept of benefit is also case specific to the patient's condition. The therapies a physician might offer a vital and healthy elder may be inappropriate for a patient of any age who is terminally ill and has, for example, a widespread bacterial infection (known as *sepsis*).

Benefit may mean very different things for the patient and the doctor, too, for their hopes for recovery are dependent on their respective expectations of outcome in the illness process. Sometimes, the patient's hopes for recovery are unrealistic and do not appropriately weigh the impact of the disease. When emotionally motivated demands are placed on a health care team to perform nonbeneficial treatment, it can be very difficult for everyone involved. Some people hold on much longer than others for one last chance to fight a disease or illness. Often, disagreement over the benefit of a therapy occurs when communications among the health provider, the patient, and the family are wanting. When expectations of outcome and ideas about useful (and nonbeneficial) treatments differ between parties, it is not surprising that conflict occurs.

Sometimes treatment will not alleviate the state of the illness but will allow the patient hours or days of consciousness that he or she will value highly. A person may want to try to survive for the birth of a grandchild, or for the celebration of a religious holiday, or to bid farewell to a relative who is traveling to see the patient. A treatment that allows continued consciousness may be valuable to the individual and therefore provide benefit as compassionate comfort care.

Will my doctor tell me if a treatment I am receiving has become nonbeneficial?

Sometimes doctors disagree about when a treatment no longer has benefit. For instance, they may weigh benefit versus burden differently. Many medications fall into this category. There may be a benefit to be gained by taking a certain drug, yet this drug therapy may have severe side effects that adversely affect the patient's quality of life. Understandably, these estimations will change with your age, your severity of illness, your short-term and long-term prognosis, and the other medical interventions that are available to you. Maintaining close communication with your doctor is the best approach to this issue.

Can I request a nonbeneficial treatment?

You may request treatments your doctor believes not to be of benefit to you, but he or she is not required to provide them. The decision will depend on how all parties concerned view a treatment. If you believe that there is a particular therapy that may help you, and if you have a reasoned understanding of what that therapy is and how it might help you, you should discuss it with your doctor. If your doctor refuses even to discuss your request, you have the right to ask for a second opinion. It may be that another doctor will disagree with your doctor, or it may be that you do not fully realize the severity of the disease or the treatment's lack of benefit. Frank discussion between you and your doctor often proves a potent antidote to miscommunication and misunderstanding.

What if my doctor refuses to provide a treatment?

The best thing to do in these circumstances is to be open and honest in your discussions with your doctor, so that your doctor knows why you are requesting the treatment. You also need to ask your doctor questions, so that you can learn why your doctor is making the decisions he or she is making. Everyone involved needs to understand the realistic course of the disease as well as the realistic chance of recovery. If there is a certain risk in a medical therapy that you are willing to accept, then it is best to discuss that with your physician early, so that he or she knows how hard you wish to fight your illness. If there is disagreement between you and your physician over the appropriateness of a therapy, then requesting a second opinion or a referral to another physician may be an advisable course of action. Your doctor may perceive an advanced disease state as a lost war, not as an ongoing battle.

Can I demand *nonbeneficial* treatment?

Demanding something *that will not benefit you* makes no medical sense, regardless of the *perceived* benefit. Perhaps the best thing to do in such circumstances is to sit down with your family and your doctor and discuss realistically what your medical options are. If you and your doctor have differing expectations regarding your medical care, it is best to address them as soon as possible.

As an example, consider an elderly man with known metastatic (widespread) colon cancer who enters the hospital with chest pain and is diagnosed as having a myocardial infarction (heart attack) due to severe coronary artery disease. His doctor believes that medical management is adequate for the patient's needs, considering his level of illness and his advanced age. His doctor is nearly certain that he will not survive an operation to bypass the diseased arteries to his heart. The doctor tells the patient that his survival is not expected to be more than several months because of the widespread cancer. The doctor does not inform him of the option of undergoing bypass surgery. The patient, however, requests that he be considered for a bypass operation "like a friend of mine just had." The doctor explains to the patient that he is not a reasonable candidate for this operation, but the patient demands (with his family's agreement) that the operation be done. The doctor refuses to perform the procedure, which he perceives to be nonbeneficial and dangerous for this patient. He volunteers the names of several doctors who might consider performing the operation. Two of the other doctors also refuse to operate; the third doctor believes that, although there is substantial risk, the operation is feasible. The operation is performed, and the patient initially does well in the surgical intensive care unit. Several hours later, however, the patient's heart arrests (stops) and cardiopulmonary resuscitation is performed. The patient's heart is restarted but he never regains consciousness. One week later, the doctor who performed the surgery explains to the family that the patient is in an irreversible comatose state, that his chances of recovery to a thinking state are nonexistent, and that the doctor is going to write a "no code" order on the chart. A *no code order* means that no attempts will be made to restart the heart or lungs if in the future they fail to function. The family is adamantly against this order and demands that it not be written in the chart. The doctor states that cardiopulmonary resuscitation (CPR) would not be beneficial and that he is willing to facilitate the transfer of the patient to another doctor. Pointing out to the family that the patient's state is grave, the doctor asks them if the patient would want to be resuscitated in his current state, with no hope of recovery. The family discuss this aspect of the patient's values and decide that he would not want such attempts made if, in the end, he would be incompetent and unable to think and speak. After these discussions among themselves and with the doctor, the family agree to have the no code order written in the chart. The patient dies the next day, after suffering another heart attack.

In this example, the patient, the patient's family, and the health care providers all had to make decisions based on their understanding of the possible benefits or lack thereof in the situation and on their beliefs, or values, as well as on the ethical principles involved. In chapter 3, we discuss the ethical principles that influence health care decisions.

3

How Ethical Principles Affect Health Care Decisions

Suppose you were ill and you needed to give your permission for or wished to refuse a treatment. What ethical grounds give you those rights?

What is autonomy?

Autonomy is the ethical principle describing the right to self-determination. It includes the right to be left alone and to make your own decisions without interference from other people. It is also the basis for your doctor's responsibility to respect you as a person and your right to make decisions about your medical care and to respect your confidentiality. The principle of autonomy (also called the principle of respect for persons) is rooted in social notions of individual freedom, constitutional rights of liberty and privacy, and U.S. court decisions made over the past several decades.

What is beneficence?

Beneficence is the principle that gives force to the physician's responsibility to attempt to benefit the patient medically while attempting to minimize harm to the patient. The foundations of this principle are more than 2,400 years old, reaching back to the time of Hippocrates. Physicians were encouraged to treat their patients by doing their best "to help, or at least to do no harm."

Why are these principles of concern to me?

The principles of autonomy and beneficence are of concern to us all. They address our ability to make decisions about our own medical care as well as our expectation that information will be given to us so we can make those decisions (within the autonomy principle), and they dictate that a physician has a responsibility to do his or her best to try to benefit the patient and protect the patient from harm (within the beneficence principle).

Do autonomy and beneficence ever come into conflict?

The doctor's beneficence-based duties toward the patient occasionally conflict with the patient's autonomy. Physicians are sometimes *paternalistic* (that is, excessively beneficent), so that they insist on helping patients whether or not the patient wants the help, or they proceed with what they regard as helpful without consulting the patient. While they may have good intentions, physicians who act paternalistically may violate the dignity and rights of the patient.

Paternalistic behavior can restrict the patient's decision-making autonomy in various ways. If the doctor were to withhold information from you to "spare" you anguish, or if you accepted a certain treatment plan as your only choice because your doctor did not inform you of available alternatives, or, in the extreme, if the physician forced a therapy upon you through coercive means, your freedom to decide would be diminished. Such behavior is professionally unethical and in some cases illegal.

Let's consider the example of a young woman who is diagnosed as having thyroid cancer and is sent to a surgeon who tells her that the tumor and surrounding tissue need to be removed. In response to the patient's question about risks, the surgeon plays down the risks of infection and bleeding and does not even mention the resulting scar and the risk of injury to the nerves going to both sides of the vocal cords. Not wanting to worry the patient, the doctor hides this information from her. After surgery, the patient discovers that one of the two nerves to the vocal cords was irreparably severed during the procedure, leaving her with speech difficulties; further, she is upset by the appearance of the scar on her neck.

This case raises the question of whether the patient would have agreed to undergo the surgery had these outcomes been explained to her. The point here is that the patient would, at the very least, have been able to prepare herself mentally for such possible adverse outcomes if the risks had been discussed with her and she chose to accept them. Paternalism in this case took the form of a doctor hiding something from a patient due to a desire to protect her from what the doctor perceived to be an unnecessary concern.

What do advance directives have to do with the principles of autonomy and beneficence?

Advance directives are designed to help you exercise your right to decide autonomously which medical therapies you want. When competent, you are always free to consent to or refuse any therapy. Therefore, you have a right to decide *before* you should become unable to speak for yourself which therapies you want attempted and which therapies you believe will not be worthwhile to you in continuing your life. The doctor's autonomy-based obligation is to follow your preferences, and the doctor's beneficence-based obligation is to offer and use only beneficial therapies (as discussed in chapter 2).

What are informed consent and informed refusal?

Informed consent is a mechanism for honoring the principle of autonomy. Because of the principle of autonomy, your doctor has a duty to tell you about your medical condition, the risks and benefits of therapies that might help you, and what might happen to you if you elect to have no treatment at all. This process is called *disclosure*. Your doctor also has the responsibility to make sure that you understand all of this information, that is, he or she must ensure *comprehension*. If you are *free of constraints* and are able to process this information and make an informed choice, then you can give an informed consent. To be free of constraints, you must be without an impairing mental condition (such as psychosis or severe dementia), without anyone trying to coerce you (for example, your doctor, a nurse, a third-party health care payer, or a family member), and able to understand your medical situation as well as the available treatment options and to use this information to make a decision. Evidence of your choice can be written, verbal, or, if you are unable to use those means, by nonverbal gestures (such as blinking your eyes or grasping a person's hand).

You might likewise give an informed refusal. You have the autonomous right to refuse any medical therapy that could be imposed on your body and to have that refusal respected by your doctor and family, as long as you have decision-making capacity when you make this decision. The necessary components of disclosure, comprehension, and freedom from constraints apply to refusal, just as they do to consent.

Informed consent should be considered a process, not an event. You engage your doctor in an active understanding of your options, and you make clear your choices to him or her. So, too, advance care planning is a process, for it begins with a decision about your advance directives, continues with detailed conversations about your values and preferences, and concludes with your linking these values and preferences to their future use in possible states of health and communicating your preferences to your doctor, proxy, family and friends. Both of these processes enable you to entrust others with making decisions on your behalf; a less thorough approach may not safeguard your autonomy.

What questions should I ask my doctor during the informed consent phase of considering a therapy?

If you are in the hospital or a doctor's office and the doctor suggests initiating a therapy for you, ask questions. Here are some examples of questions to ask if the doctor has not already volunteered the information:

What is my medical condition called?
What are the implications of this condition?
What will happen to me as time goes on?
What is my short-term prognosis? What is my long-term prognosis?
What is the therapy called?
What does the therapy do?
How does the therapy work?
How invasive is the therapy?
How long will I have to continue the therapy?
What is the benefit to be gained by using this therapy?
What are the risks of this therapy?
What other therapies may possibly be beneficial to me?
What would happen if I didn't treat this condition?
What are the chances this therapy will help me?
Will I (or my proxy) be free to stop this therapy if it does not help me?

How much will this therapy cost?

How will this therapy burden my family (financially, physically) if a prolonged recovery time is required?

Can a person who has dementia, mental retardation, or mental illness give informed consent?

Any adult person who can understand the nature of his or her disease, appreciate his or her options for treatments, and make a voluntary, unconstrained choice is capable of giving a legally valid informed consent or refusal. Further, any person who is able to give informed consent is also able to prepare an advance directive. A person's capacity to give informed consent may vary over time, however; today someone may be unable to understand or freely choose, while tomorrow that person may be able to do so. An example of such a circumstance is the patient with early Alzheimer's disease, whose ability to give informed consent can vary from day to day or even hour to hour. In our experience, persons with mental illness or mental retardation, as well as those with early dementia, may be able to give valid consent to an advance directive, depending on the ability of the patient.

Can minors give informed consent?

Yes, to a certain extent, minors can participate in their consent. As children grow up, they mature in both physical and intellectual ways. A boy at 7 may be able to contribute his perceptions of whether he wants to be treated for an illness, although his parents will ultimately be responsible for the decision. As a child matures through adolescence, the capacity to reason, weigh alternatives, and make choices generally increases. Hence, the same boy at 17 may be able to give informed consent, if his state's laws permit it.

Current laws governing the execution of living wills and durable powers of attorney exclude minors. But, while minors of a certain age (the age differs by state) cannot sign a binding power of attorney or living will, they *can* express their wishes about life-sustaining medical therapies, by discussing the issues with their parents and their doctor.

How is informed consent important to my doctor?

The physician's duty to respect you as a person and to solicit your informed consent guarantees your rights to make your own choices and to expect that they will be honored. Although physicians may know more about your condition and your treatment options than you do, you have the right to be given all information relevant to making your own decisions about medical treatments. The physician's responsibility to ensure an informed consent thereby offsets the possibility of paternalistic coercion that could force a particular decision.

Regardless of the physician's perception of his or her obligation to make you better again, you have a right to refuse medical treatment. However, the physician also has a professional autonomy.

What does the physician's professional autonomy have to do with me?

Physicians have the right not to be forced to violate their own moral, professional, or religious codes, provided they do not abandon a patient. If you go to a doctor who has strong views that conflict with your choices, he or she has a right to withdraw from your case, as long as responsibility for your care is transferred to another doctor (this right is recognized in most advance directive legislation). All of us, including physicians, have values and moral beliefs that underlie our attitudes and influence our behaviors.

What is justice?

Justice is the principle of dealing fairly and equitably with people. Sometimes, in the context of medicine, justice is related to the allocation of limited resources. Broadly interpreted, however, justice encompasses fair and equitable treatment of persons under whatever system is being considered.

How is justice important in medicine?

Justice has become increasingly important in medicine as the money available for health care increasingly seems insufficient to meet people's medical needs. As a result, constraints have been placed on hospitals to curb the amount of money spent on health care. The U.S. government has started regulating the length of hospital stays for procedures and for administration of medical therapies. The government implemented these programs in an attempt to distribute funds to hospitals more equitably, to provide for the health care needs of more people.

Can justice interfere with other principles?

Justice-based concerns of trying to share the cost of health care more equitably could interfere with other ethical principles if they influenced the physician's or hospital's decision to hospitalize a patient. Treatment decisions based solely on economic considerations—rather than on the patient's benefit—would be ethically suspect. On the other hand, sometimes "high-tech," high-cost therapies are not medically justifiable because the chance of gaining any benefit is extremely remote. For instance, every time you get a tension (or muscle contraction) headache, your doctor shouldn't request a computer-enhanced scan of the brain (and neither should you). To do so would enormously drive up the costs of medical care for everyone while exposing you to radiation and likely not finding anything wrong anyway.

Where do I fit in this picture?

As a patient, you have certain rights that must be respected. You have the right to receive sound medical therapy and the right to refuse that therapy. Further, you have the right to expect that no one will coerce individual medical practitioners or health care facilities into changing the practice of medicine in a way that adversely affects the delivery of health care. You fit in as a consumer safeguarding your own interests within the health care system.

4

THE VALUE

OF VALUES

Suppose you want to consider your future medical decisions. What kinds of personal values and beliefs would be helpful in exploring these matters and discussing them with your loved ones and your doctor?

What are values?

Values are the beliefs we hold that allow us to frame our perspective of life from day to day. They can be religious, cultural, or philosophical in nature. Values develop as we grow up within our families, our communities, and society.

Why are values important?

Values are important because they help to formulate the decisions we may make in our lives. The values we hold guide our opinions of the world around us and our place in that world. By examining our own values, we can better understand *how* we perceive the world and *why* we perceive it as we do.

What are attitudes?

Attitudes describe the feelings we have about the things we encounter in life. Attitudes are based on our emotional reactions and intellectual reflections. Positive or negative attitudes toward challenges, setbacks, and success, for example, are part of the value system we have developed. We develop these attitudes in response to our experiences with the world. The projection of our attitudes in our behavior toward others reflects the values that we hold.

How do values and attitudes interact?

Values and attitudes interact and reflect each other. Values help to form attitudes. If we hold values that reflect a certain belief system, our attitudes will likely also reflect those values. The interaction between our values and our attitudes, often not even recognized by us, influences our behavior.

What are behaviors?

Behaviors are the means by which we demonstrate our values and attitudes. Behaviors come in the form of action and in the form of inaction. The way in which we conduct ourselves in the world and with those around us—this is our behavior.

How do values and attitudes affect behaviors?

Values and attitudes act as a catalyst for the way we behave toward others. For example, if we hold values and attitudes that are critical of a particular action, we probably will not engage in that action. Likewise, if our values and attitudes include a belief that it is worthwhile to do a particular thing, our behavior will probably reflect that fact. We do not always behave in accord with our attitudes, however. Sometimes we engage in actions that do not necessarily "fit in" with the attitudes we project; for example, a conservative, practical person may impulsively buy a sports car.

Are medical values different from other values?

Medical values are a subset of the other values that we hold. Medical values are applied to a specific part of life: medical issues. For example, we may broadly value being free as individuals; a corresponding medical value would address our wish to have freedom and respect shown to us when we make medical decisions for ourselves.

How do medical values play a role in my attitudes and behaviors, such as advance directive decisions?

Your values will be reflected in your attitudes, and these, in turn, will direct your behavior. For example, if you value being informed about your medical care and if you value your freedom to choose future medical therapies, these values will be reflected in your attitudes toward your health care, such as a desire for independence or not to be in pain. Along with your reflections on past personal experiences and those of family members, these attitudes will contribute to your behavior concerning your health care decisions as well as to how you behave when you interact with your doctor and in your current interest in signing an advance directive.

So, are medical values somehow linked to advance directives?

Research conducted by Dr. David Doukas demonstrated that certain medical values are related to the formulation of advance directives. In two recent investigations, the selection of values and advance directives was studied in two different populations: a multigenerational population and an outpatient population of well adults. Participants in these studies were asked to rank their agreement with a variety of important values in medical care as well as the desirability of several medical therapies listed in the Values History (see the Appendix). In both studies, patient values about imposing burdens on the family were inversely correlated with the preferences toward life-sustaining medical therapies for terminal illness. In other words, the more intense the person's concern about family burden (such as being a financial or physical burden on other members of the family), the less likely it was that the person wanted life-sustaining medical therapies. These findings may reflect a pragmatic concern by patients about pain-related and burden-related issues.

How do I apply these values when considering advance directives?

Research by many other medical ethics scholars has also been helpful in arguing for describing one's wishes in the future health scenarios that might occur. Granted, no one can tell what sort of medical state one may be in in five, ten, or twenty years. The best way to apply one's values in this process is to have discussions with others about how one wants to be treated in the case of *terminal illness and incapacity, irreversible coma, persistent vegetative state,* and *end-stage dementia.* These discussions can serve as touchstones for determining one's medical preferences. Bringing your values to each of these potential circumstances can help you identify what you would want, and making these wishes known to your loved ones can ease their decision making on your behalf. Conscious application of your values provides the best avenue for fruitful discussion and for easing the angst that comes with such discussions, and it is most likely to illuminate a path of respect for patient autonomy.

Should I discuss my medical values with my family?

We believe that an essential part of advance care planning is discussing your values with your family. Discussing your values and your medical preferences with your family allows them to understand the context of your medical values and decisions, to be more accepting should these preferences need to be carried out, and to be better surrogates for you if you cannot communicate. These discussions allow for an open exchange of ideas between you and your family, so there is no chance for a misunderstanding about why you wish to sign an advance directive.

When a family member acts as a proxy, there is a presumption that the family member has an intimate knowledge of the patient's values and preferences, or is at least trusted enough to be named as proxy in a durable power of attorney for health care. Such knowledge is based on a relationship of trust and understanding, in which values and medical preferences are discussed. If such in-depth discussions do not take place, the patient may someday be done a grave disservice. (For information about the various values that can be discussed, see chapter 6.)

Is there anyone else with whom I ought to consider discussing my medical values?

You definitely should have discussions with the person you are likely to select as your proxy, or health care agent, who may or may not be a family member. It is critically important for you to discuss your values and preferences regarding medical care with your proxy, to make sure the person understands your values and preferences. It is also essential to identify any problems, ambiguities, or conflicts between you and your proxy. Also, discussions with your religious or spiritual adviser can help you clarify or better articulate your religious and philosophical values. Such discussions should be for the purpose of helping you discover your own values, not to allow someone else to tell you what values you should have. This process is introspective and reflective—the answers need to come from within you.

Will my doctor find it helpful to be acquainted with my values?

Yes. Information about your values will give your doctor insight into the factors that contributed to your decision to sign an advance directive and the choices reflected in it. By knowing about the values and attitudes you hold, your doctor may better understand your decisions. Even your doctor cannot imagine all the many scenarios of illness or predict which illnesses you will encounter (including in what way you might become terminally ill or otherwise unable to recover). If you have discussed your *general* medical values and attitudes with your doctor, and then someday you're unable to talk for yourself or express yourself, your doctor will be better able, with the assistance of your family, to interpret your preferences on medical treatment in a broader light.

When should I discuss my values with others?

There is no "best time" to discuss your values with either your family or your doctor; nor is there any good reason to delay doing so. Given the unpredictability of life, we advise you to discuss your values, in the context of your advance directives, with your family and doctor as soon as possible, so that other people will be familiar with your medical values if you become unable to make decisions.

Will my values change over time?

It is very likely that your values will change over your lifetime. We are all dynamic creatures, and as we experience new positive and negative events, our values change. How much they change—

whether just slightly or dramatically—depends upon how firmly we believe in our value system when we encounter such events. As a result, it is wise to update any method of values assessment periodically (we recommend doing this at least every twelve months, maybe around your birthday, for instance), as well as when any major health changes occur. This allows you to reflect on the latest events in your life and to examine what effect they have had on your value system.

If my values will change, why should I explore them now?

Thinking about these values now can help you prepare to make future decisions and help you make your advance directives. People tend to put off thinking about advance directives, but since, as we've said, it's impossible to predict when a life-threatening illness or accident might occur, we recommend that, if you haven't already done so, you start thinking about your medical values now, and communicating them to loved ones. Communicating these values is particularly helpful when the communication is in writing. These decisions can be formalized using a living will, a durable power of attorney for health care, and a Values History. We turn to the first two of these advance directives in the next chapter.

5

How Advance

Directives Work

Suppose you are interested in making a declaration about medical treatments that you want or do not want. What do you need to know about advance directives before you sign one?

Why were advance directives developed?

As technology has advanced over the years and has become better able to keep people alive longer, many people have wanted a way to say, "Enough is enough." Indeed, some people have voiced the fear that they will be sustained on medical machines and therapies against their will. Advance directives were first developed to allow people to tell their doctors and family what kinds of medical therapies they wish to refuse in case of terminal illness.

Competent adults have the right to consent to or refuse any medical therapy. Advance directives provide a way for a person to state in advance which medical treatments the person desires and which are not desired under certain circumstances, and then to have these wishes carried out if the person later is unable to make or express a choice when a health care decision must be made.

When were advance directives developed?

Living wills were developed in the mid-1970s, beginning with the 1976 Natural Death Act in California and eventually spreading across the country to nearly every state. Even states without a living will statute still allow you to make a written declaration on end-of-life treatment.

The durable power of attorney for health care, which allows for the appointment of a surrogate decision maker for health care (also called an *agent* or *proxy*), was developed more recently. Durable powers of attorney *for health care* have been legalized explicitly by statute in most states, while general durable powers of attorney can be used in all states.

What is the purpose of advance directives?

Both living wills and durable powers of attorney for health care allow a person to express health care preferences that are to be implemented if he or she is terminally ill (in many states, also if in a persistent vegetative state) and unable to communicate these preferences. Also, durable powers of attorney allow a person to relate what he or she wants done in the event of any future incapacity. The foundation of a person's ability to sign a living will or durable power of attorney is informed consent. As discussed in chapter 3, informed consent is the autonomous right of the person to approve or refuse a medical therapy or treatment plan that has been offered or recommended to him or her. Informed consent requires disclosure of information about the therapy, understanding of that information and of one's medical condition, freedom from pressure to decide one way or another, and an ability to use this information to make a decision.

What is a terminal illness?

A terminal illness is generally understood to be an illness that will inevitably lead to death, despite medical intervention. Medical intervention may prolong the life of the person, but the disease process continues, so medical intervention can also prolong dying.

How is persistent vegetative state defined?

A *persistent vegetative state* is an irreversible neurological condition in which a person can no longer respond knowingly to others or communicate with them in any way but is capable of breathing on his or her own. A person in a persistent vegetative state has suffered damage to the brain from trauma or lack of oxygen that impairs the person's ability to think, feel, reason, and communicate. A person in a persistent vegetative state may exhibit reflex responses to certain stimuli and may go through what appear to be sleep and wake cycles, but the person will not be able to perceive (that is cannot see or hear) what is going on around him or her and will not be able to communicate with others.

A persistent vegetative state is different from an *irreversible coma*. A person in an irreversible coma is permanently in a sleep-like state and has no wakeful episodes. The person is not able to communicate and does not have sleep-wake cycles. An irreversible coma is the result of irreparable damage to massive areas of the brain caused by oxygen deprivation.

A *reversible coma* is usually the result of acute, but less severe, injury to the brain from trauma (an automobile accident, for example) or from a drug overdose. The person will eventually "come out" of this kind of coma.

What is incapacity?

In the context of the topic of this book, incapacity means an inability to understand the treatment choices presented, to appreciate the implications of the available alternatives, and to make and communicate a decision about health care. Incapacity can be temporary and reversible (for example, a result of illness or injury) or long lasting and irreversible (for example, in end-stage dementia).

Decision-making capacity is sometimes (though not always) defined in state laws governing health care decisions and advance directives. Usually, before an advance directive becomes operational, one or two physicians must examine the person and certify that he or she lacks the capacity to make a decision.

How is incapacity related to advance directives?

You have the right to make your own health care decisions as long as you possess the decision-making capacity to do so. Whether or not you have signed a living will or a durable power of attorney for health care, when you have the capacity to make decisions (or if you lose that capacity but later regain it), you have the right to make these decisions yourself.

It is only when you lose your decision-making capacity that advance directives may become critical in your health care. If you become incapacitated and are thus unable to make health care decisions, then an advance directive can speak for you. On the other hand, if you become incapacitated and do not have an advance directive, your family and your doctor may be forced to make a decision for you, based on what they know of your general attitudes and values. Under some circumstances, a court may have to make decisions for you or authorize a family member or friend to do so. Making medical decisions for an incapacitated person based on his or her formal expression of medical values and preferences in an advance directive is far easier than making such decisions based on general impressions of that person's life values.

Who can sign an advance directive?

Any adult person of sound mind who has the capacity to formulate an informed consent can sign an advance directive. (Some states currently limit the right of pregnant patients to refuse certain treatments, in order to protect the developing fetus, although some experts believe that this restriction is legally flawed.) Soundness of mind is necessary because you must understand the importance and implications of an advance directive in order for it to be valid. The witnesses will attest that you signed voluntarily. The voluntary nature of the signature indicates that you were not forced into making the decision, that your decision was not made in a frivolous or coerced manner, and that you were not in a mentally unbalanced state when you made the decision.

What might motivate me to sign a living will or a durable power of attorney for health care?

An individual's motivation for signing a living will or a durable power of attorney for health care is the desire (and the right) to record what sort of therapies he or she would want and not want if he or she were ever unable to voice a consent or refusal. The decision to sign an advance directive is relevant for both young and older adults, as accident or illness can strike at any age. These documents also allow the person who has a known illness to declare which therapies in his or her current medical condition would be acceptable and which should not be started or continued in the future, should the illness lead to decision-making incapacity. Advance directives give the person the opportunity to voice personal values and goals in a well-reasoned statement that allows the physician to understand the person's rationale for choosing to accept or refuse such care. Not making such a declaration may jeopardize your ability to be treated in the manner of your choosing if you should someday be unable to speak for yourself. It may also put your loved ones in the difficult position of selecting therapies for you based on their guesses about what you would choose. Also, if you don't have an advance directive and you someday become unable to communicate, you may be subjected to medical therapies that you do not want.

With the passage of the Patient Self-Determination Act, patients will be given more opportunities than in the past to learn about advance directives. The problem with the act lies in the circumstances under which it is carried out. That is, unless you are enrolled in a health maintenance organization, the forms will probably not be given to you (unless you obtain them on your own) until you are admitted to a hospital, nursing home, hospice, or other health agency. That may be too late, however, because you may not be able to fill out an advance directive at that time; you may be unconscious, or you may be in too much pain. We urge you to sign an advance directive *now*, while you are thinking about your values for medical care. (The web links you need to complete your advance directives are included in the Appendix.)

Whom should I choose as my proxy or agent for my durable power of attorney for health care?

You can select any adult who you think would faithfully represent your values and preferences regarding medical therapies. This person should be well acquainted with your values and preferences. While many people choose a relative to serve as their proxy, a proxy can be anyone (a spouse, a friend, a significant other) who can accurately convey your wishes to a health care team if you are unable to speak for yourself. (There is more on this subject in chapter 7.)

Before you sign a durable power of attorney which specifies the person who will serve as your agent, you must ask that person whether he or she is willing to do so, since the proxy assumes a serious responsibility on agreeing to convey your instructions to your doctor. The proxy designate can be assured that you will not be charging him or her with making decisions based on his or her own personal judgment and values, however. Rather, the proxy is responsible for serving as a conduit between you and your doctor. The decisions are actually coming from you (through your stated or recorded values and preferences) and not from the proxy. Also, your proxy should be reassured that he or she is not financially responsible for your care on the basis of this designation (he or she may be responsible owing to another relationship to you, like marriage if your proxy is your spouse).

It is also important that you and your proxy periodically review your health care values and preferences, so that he or she can remain updated. You can take the initiative to see that this happens.

Can my doctor serve as my proxy?

No. Your doctor cannot serve as your proxy because of the conflict of interest that may arise between the physician's role of healing and the fulfillment of the patient's autonomous preferences. Also, in many states, your doctor is prohibited by law from serving as your proxy.

Are the forms for living wills and durable powers of attorney for health care the same in all states?

Not exactly, as there are differences in the way state legislatures have written some of the statutes. These differences may affect both the form and the content of advance directives. You must learn about *your own state's laws* regarding the living will and the durable power of attorney in order to understand how the documents are used in your state. (Again, see the Appendix for your state's version, available free through the Internet.)

Common features of durable powers of attorney for health care are: identification of the person (or persons) appointed to act as your agent (or agents) if you are incapacitated (whether by accident or illness), the ability to apply this empowerment to all medical decision making on your behalf, and the ability to provide detailed instructions that you want your agent to follow if you are unable to speak for yourself.

Common features of living will statutes are: the right to include personalized advance instructions for circumstances of a future terminal illness with incapacity or a persistent vegetative state, the need for one or two physicians to certify that the patient is in such a medical state prior to implementation, the requirement of the doctor either to follow the provisions of a valid living will or to transfer care of the patient, the requirement of the doctor to incorporate a known living will into the medical record, the requirement to have two witnesses to the patient's signing of the document, and a release of the doctor and health facility from liability for following the living will.

Some states have passed living will statutes that do not allow for the withdrawal or withholding of artificial nutrition and hydration (although some state courts have declared that limitation unconstitutional). Some states allow for family consent or oral declarations of a living will (nevertheless, we recommend that everyone provide a *written* statement, which provides portability and verification). Many living will laws require doctors who cannot carry out the living will to transfer the patient to another doctor who will honor it. Some states explicitly allow for the honoring of a living will signed in another state, while others do not address that issue. (People who live part-time in two or more states may want to sign a declaration that is valid for both states or sign separate living wills for each of the states.)

Your own state's versions of the durable power of attorney for health care and the living will are likely to be worded slightly differently from other states' and will cover different aspects of health care. That's why it's best to obtain a copy of your own state's advance directives.

Despite minor differences, the forms are so similar between states that a document executed in one state is likely to be honored in another state, to the extent permitted under local laws. But, again, to be safe, it's best to obtain a document that has been approved for use in *your* state. (Instructions for obtaining these forms are provided in chapter 8 and the Appendix.)

Do I have to consult anyone before I sign?

No, there is no requirement that you consult with anyone before you sign an advance directive. Nevertheless, we believe you should review your values, attitudes, and preferences with your physician before you sign an advance directive, so that you're certain that you have an adequate understanding of the consequences of your decisions.

Through discussion, you and your trusted family and/or friends and your doctor will gain a much better understanding of what you are consenting to or refusing, and why. In this way, you will be making informed choices, rather than independently signing an advance directive without having the benefit of adequate knowledge and reflection. At the same time, your doctor will better understand your motivations for making the decisions you make and for signing an advance directive in the first place.

Is there a possibility that my doctor won't know enough about advance directives to help me?

It is possible. In a 1991 nationwide survey, Dr. Doukas and his colleagues asked more than 400 family physicians about their knowledge of, clinical use of, and personal use of the living will. Information about physician-initiated and patient-initiated discussions of the living will was also elicited. Physicians were asked to give their view as to the appropriateness of having a living will and to identify their sources of information about living wills. Physicians are less likely to initiate living will discussions in general (they are waiting for you to start them), and they are less likely to start conversations if they are not familiar with living wills or are afraid that the tone of the discussion will worry you or your family. This information about some physicians' attitudes demonstrates again the necessity for patients to be insistent when it comes to a discussion of advance directives.

Of the respondents in the survey, 95 percent reported being aware of the living will, 69 percent reported using living wills in caring for patients, and 71 percent of the physicians reported that their patients had come to them to initiate conversations about a living will. The more doctors know about living wills, the more they seem to value and use them, both professionally and personally.

When asked how they had learned of the living will, 56 percent of the physicians cited their patients; 47 percent, the medical literature; and 31 percent, the media. It appears that patients have more influence on doctors than we realize! This study shows that your doctor may be much more likely to discuss advance directives if *you bring up* the use of advance directives during an office visit (and may be less likely to do so otherwise). So, yes, you should bring up advance directives with your doctor, and if needed bring materials so you can help him or her understand why this is important to you in your future health care. Just as you have heard much about the recent Schiavo case, so have doctors, and they undoubtedly will be sensitized to the issues and more willing to engage you in discussions about advance directives. No doctor would ever want the fate of the Schiavo/Schindler family to visit the home of any of his or her own patients.

Do I need witnesses when I sign an advance directive?

Yes. On the advance directive forms you will find a description of the intent of the form: to stipulate that you will forgo treatment if terminally ill (on the living will) and that you transfer decision-making authority to a proxy if incapacitated (on the durable power of attorney for health care). Below this description are lines for your signature and the date and lines for witnesses to sign *at the same time*. For both the living will and the durable power of attorney for health care, witnesses must see you sign the document before they sign it. In some states, a notary public's acknowledgment of someone's signature can substitute for witnesses.

Why are witnesses required?

Witnessing shows that the person who signed did so knowingly and freely. The signatures of witnesses show that you, not someone else, actually signed the directive, and they may also serve as testimonials to your competence at the time of the signing. Because it is witnessed, the document is far less likely to be challenged in the future (again, this depends on state law).

Can anyone serve as a witness?

A witness should not be a relative, a health care provider, an employee of a health care provider, or an heir of the person whose directive is being formalized. These provisions guard against any possible conflict of interest.

How long are advance directives valid?

Several state statutes originally required that living wills be renewed periodically. Now, all states that allow a living will by statute have revised those laws, so that once a living will is signed, it remains valid unless the patient revokes it. Durable powers of attorney for health care also last indefinitely, unless the person writing the document decides to limit the time during which it will be effective.

What happens if I want to withdraw or change my advance directive?

You can revoke a living will or durable power of attorney for health care by destroying it or by writing the word *void* across it. You always have the right to revoke an advance directive. Revoking a living will means that you *do* want life-sustaining therapies begun or continued if you are terminally ill or persistently vegetative. In most states, even mentally incapacitated patients with advance directives must be treated if they request it. You can also change the person to whom you give decision-making authority or modify your instructions. You can execute a new advance directive and make it clear that this document supersedes all previously executed directives. Signing an advance directive today does not mean that you can't change your mind later. You *can*.

What challenging issues occur in the use of advance directives?

One issue is that the advance directive may not be relevant to a clinical situation that happens to you, so the directive may not be useful in that situation. There are also instances in which the instructions provided in advance directives may be too vague to be understood. Expressions such as "Let me please die if my brain is not functioning" do not provide as much guidance as more specific wording does.

The advance directive may become outdated, no longer expressing the patient's preferences because their values or health circumstances have changed over time. Also, a proxy or agent designated in the durable power of attorney for health care may not truly know the wishes, preferences, values, and religious beliefs of the patient. This problem can arise when ongoing communication is not part of the advance directive process.

The designated proxy (or designated agent) may not be up to making an appropriate decision, may feel ill prepared to make an appropriate decision, or may feel pressured about "having to make a decision." Although the physician can encourage the patient to discuss specific issues with the proxy, the patient may want to rely solely on the trust that he or she has in a proxy who is a loved one.

A frequent problem is that someone designates another person as proxy but never talks to the proxy about what they want. When the person later is ill and needs decisions made in his or her behalf, the proxy is left holding the "decision-making bag" without a clear understanding of what the person would have wanted done. Specific and repeated *conversations* about what drives one's health care values and preferences are essential in order for the proxy to make decisions for you later. Without such discussions, the paper the proxy holds will have far less meaning.

Another challenge in the use of advance directives occurs when there is an emergency situation outside of an institutional setting and the proxy cannot be located. There also are situations in which a physician fails to involve the proxy in decision making. In addition, the proxy may find him- or herself having to advocate for the patient's values and preferences, which may be difficult in a complex situation unfolding in a hospital or nursing facility and with the possibility of divergent health care professional values.

Can competent patients allow their proxy to make decisions for them?

Patients should never be forced to make health care decisions. In cases where patients do not want to decide for themselves, a durable power of attorney can be written so it takes effect immediately and stays in effect after incapacity. Any patient (whether well or ill—including chronically ill) may say to the proxy or doctor that he or she does not want to discuss these health care issues, and may ask that the proxy be consulted about any issue that comes up. While patients have a right to *waive* their right to make decisions, it needs to be made clear that waiving this right makes future proxy decision making more challenging. Also, patients need to know that they can always reengage in their health care decision making, even if they previously waived their right. The use of advance directives is far more helpful for patients, their loved ones, and their doctors when the directive and the proxy can be clear about what the patient wants or does not want done in terms of health care. Therefore, discussing *both* one's values and one's preferences is an extremely helpful part of advance care planning.

What does the Terri Schiavo case teach us?

The Schiavo case teaches us that all of these concerns about advance directives need to be addressed. There are three ways to do this:

1. Execute an advance directive.
2. Have meaningful discussions with your doctor and your selected proxy on what values and preferences you hold for future states of terminal illness and incapacity. We owe it to our proxy to engage in a meaningful discussion-based process regarding what we want and do not want and why, so that person can best represent us someday. Then review your values and health care preferences periodically with your physician and proxy and other loved ones whom you trust.
3. Make sure that your family and other loved ones know who your proxy is and that your proxy knows whom you want him or her to talk to in future cases of incapacity—and whom *not* to talk to as well.

This period of raised public consciousness after the Schiavo cases affords us all the opportunity to make a paradigm shift of our own—to begin discussing our values and preferences with our family and doctors so that future decisions can be made appropriately for us if we cannot make decisions for ourselves. We believe that we all have a responsibility to ourselves and our physician, proxy, family members, and other loved ones to have in-depth conversations about what we want in our future health care, whom we want to speak on our behalf, how our family plays a role in this process, and how we want our doctor to respond. This is a tall order indeed, but our ability to make these values and preferences clear in advance will safeguard our future interests during medical care.

Can a relative or acquaintance challenge the authority of an advance directive?

A problem may occur if the patient has asked that life-prolonging treatments be discontinued and someone else questions that request. Suppose that the proxy, the entire family, and the hospital ethics committee are in agreement with the patient's wishes as expressed in his living will. A cousin from a distant state, let's call him "Cousin Bob," who has not seen the patient for more than seven years, arrives and insists that everything possible be done to maintain his cousin's life. Is this response one of guilt or grief? Cousin Bob then threatens legal action against the doctor and the hospital. If this advance directive was properly executed and has been discussed with the patient's doctor, and possibly with the patient's lawyer, the physician can feel certain that he or she is doing the right thing in following the wishes expressed in the advance directive. The sensitive response here is to acknowledge Bob's grief but point out that abiding by a legally expressed autonomous preference is most respectful of the patient's dignity.

When a properly completed directive is available, it is the physician's duty to write medical orders that reflect the patient's wishes and instructions. It would be beneficial to communicate these orders and the patient's instructions to other physicians and nurses who may have occasion to care for the patient. The patient's family, too, should be informed that the treatment underway fulfills what the patient had requested.

The authority of proxies is also sometimes challenged, but it is just as legally sound as the instructions in a directive. There is the possibility that a proxy's decisions are based on self-interest: Could the proxy benefit from the patient's premature death, or from a prolongation of life, such as keeping the patient in a persistent vegetative state? Most people involved with advance health care planning believe that such acts of self-interest occur infrequently. Physicians and family can feel comfortable that the proxy's decisions are in harmony with what the patient truly requested.

6

THE VALUES HISTORY:
DEFINING YOUR
HEALTH CARE VALUES

Suppose you are thinking about having a living will and/or a durable power of attorney, but they don't seem sufficient to record what you wish to say on this subject. Is there any additional way for you to provide your loved ones and your doctor with more detailed information about and understanding of your wishes regarding specific approaches to care and treatment?

What is the Values History?

The "Values History," an advance directive form developed by Dr. David Doukas and Dr. Laurence McCullough, is designed to enhance current advance directives. (Dr. Edmund Pellegrino coined the term *value history* in the early 1980s to describe the discussions that might take place that would enable a doctor to elicit the values that are important to a patient's health care decisions, and the naming of the Values History instrument has been an enduring tribute to Dr. Pellegrino's pioneering efforts.) The Values History by Doukas and McCullough (see Appendix of this book) is intended to *supplement* a living will or durable power of attorney by stimulating a person's thinking about specific medical values and eliciting from people statements concerning the values that would be important to them in the event of a terminal illness or if they were in a persistent vegetative state. Further, the Values History contains explicit advance directive statements regarding many medical therapies. An individual can complete these statements and be assured that the document will clearly state his or her wishes to family members and health care personnel.

This document allows the person to specify for each treatment the person's acceptance, rejection, or—a third choice—the person's willingness to have the health care team attempt a trial of that intervention. In a *trial of intervention,* a therapy is carried out for a specified period or as long as it takes to determine either that a specific benefit will be gained through the therapy or that the treatment is without benefit.

The Values History is a valuable tool to help you in the advance directive process. We believe that using the Values History by Doukas and McCullough has the following advantage: by prompting you to reflect *meaningfully* on your *medical values* and by preparing you to formulate *specific* advance directives, the Values History allows you to express your values more meaningfully and more specifically than other documents do. At the same time, the Values History facilitates your reflection on these important values through a series of questions and statements. These values and preferences are then discussed with your proxy and with those family members and loved ones whom you want to be part of your future medical decisions, so that your autonomy can be better respected through enhanced communication. This values conversation may be pivotal to your own end-of-life care.

What kinds of questions does the Values History ask?

The Values History helps you express your values by, first, inquiring which is more important to you at the end of your life: a good quality of life, regardless of whether that life is shortened, or a longer life, regardless of the quality of that life. This choice is fundamental in terms of medical values.

The Values History next lists many values having to do with such issues as your ability to communicate, your desire to have your doctor carry out your wishes, and your wish to avoid placing various burdens on your family due to your illness. The Values History asks you to circle those values that are most meaningful to you. You are also encouraged to add other values that are important to you and to expand on your previously voiced values. You then are asked to say how and why these values would be relevant to you in case of terminal illness with incapacity, dementia, persistent vegetative state, or irreversible coma.

Finally, the Values History turns to a series of medical interventions that are possible and assesses your preferences regarding these interventions in the above circumstances. Both acute interventions (such as cardiopulmonary resuscitation and ventilator use) and chronic interventions (such as feeding tube use and dialysis) are considered in the Values History. We think it is crucial for you and your doctor to discuss these therapies and how they might be important for you. (Chapter 8 describes the steps involved in completing the Values History.)

How can the Values History help me?

The Values History can be helpful to you if you have strong feelings about protecting yourself from pain or protecting your family against harm or burden, if you have concerns about voicing your health care decisions, or if you have preferences about how you want your physician to comply with your desires. By listing these values, you can clarify for the health care team the values that underlie the advance directives you select.

The Values History can also help those who may, in the future, need to interpret the intent of your previously signed advance directives. By elaborating on your medical values and directives regarding treatment, it enables others to carry out your wishes better by providing a richer context for your values and directives.

No living will or durable power of attorney can cover all medical contingencies. Remember, the Values History is intended to *supplement* a living will or durable power of attorney for health care that you have already signed. The Values History gives these documents fuller meaning, so that unforeseen events can be addressed with greater understanding of your medical values and directives.

How does the Values History help me discuss my treatment preferences and values with my doctor and family?

Physicians and families can act as sounding boards, helping you think through decisions on advance directives. The Values History encourages you to hold these discussions, in that it asks questions about your own individual values. The questioning and answering that goes on between you and your physician, and you and your family, increases everyone's ability to understand your feelings, values, and attitudes as well as the implications of your treatment decisions. The values and preferences that you put into your Values History should reflect a meaningful ongoing conversation that you have had with your proxy, your doctor, your friends, and your family. These persons then will understand the fuller context of your values and the meanings of your preferences; you, too, will benefit from their questions about these values and preferences because they give you an opportunity to be still clearer about your wishes.

The discussions you have now and in the future with your doctor may one day be very important for your health care. These discussions will help your doctor understand the circumstances of illness under which you would want your advance directives carried out. Holding these discussions frankly and openly helps avoid misunderstandings about your wishes regarding life-sustaining therapy. Please understand that *merely filling out a form* will *never replace* deep conversations about what in life drives your decisions and shades your preferences about accepting or refusing treatment. The conversations about *what* holds meaning to you is essential to this process.

Are there legal barriers to the use of the Values History?

The Values History can be an important asset in the informed consent or refusal process for both ethical and legal reasons. It has standing ethically under the right of any competent adult to make an informed and free medical treatment decision. It also has legal standing to the extent that nearly all states allow you to add specific instructions to your living will and durable power of attorney. In these states, patient health care statements that are attached to their advance directives apply to future health care with the same legal force. It is intended that the Values History be attached as an addendum to a valid signed living will **and** durable power of attorney for health care (using a metaphorical "belt and suspenders" to help make sure that you are protected). Including a Values History makes clearer what you want and do not want under what circumstances, and who should then safeguard the implementation of those wishes in the future.

A few states currently limit some of the types of decisions you might make (such as refusing nutrition and hydration) in your

Values History, but you should state your preferences anyway, as such limitations can change over time. It is also possible that you will be in a different jurisdiction when a decision must be made about your care.

Besides legal barriers, is there anything else that might obstruct the implementation of my preferences in my Values History?

Sometimes doctors and family members attempt to interfere with the implementation of a person's preferences as stated in an advance directive. If your doctor is not willing to carry out your advance directives, he or she should promptly arrange to transfer your care to another doctor. If your health care proxy feels that your doctor is not carrying out your wishes, he or she ought to arrange for your care to be transferred. When there is no advance directive and there is a division between family members, as occurred with the Schiavo case, then litigation may result, if there is no middle ground for mediation.

When a family tries to obstruct fulfillment of advance directives, it is usually because of a conflict of intent (usually they want treatment that the patient has declined) or conflict of interest (this is discussed in chapter 7). Sometimes it is difficult for a family to know how a patient would view a particular medical condition; they may disagree about how to interpret or apply an advance directive. If this happens, then the doctor and family members can seek the advice and counsel of an ethics committee, which almost all hospitals have.

Do I have only two options? Must I either agree to a treatment or refuse it?

Your advance directives regarding health care need not be absolute. In the Values History, you are free to voice your preferences to specific directives in a method of *limited consent* known as a *trial of intervention.* A trial of intervention allows you to designate a length of time after which you would want a treatment stopped or a circumstance under which you would want a treatment stopped.

In a trial of intervention, a treatment is initiated and then monitored to determine whether it will be of benefit. If the treatment doesn't help after a *time period that you set,* it can be discontinued. For example, if you designate a trial of intervention to allow the use of a ventilator for two weeks, and if the ventilator proves to be nonbeneficial during this time and recovery is deemed hopeless, your doctor could then honor your wish to discontinue its use. Alternatively, you could designate a trial of intervention whereby the therapy is continued, *provided that it is medically beneficial* to you (regardless of the duration of the intervention). If the treatment is initiated and, after a period considered reasonable by the physician and your proxy, it has rendered you no benefit, the treatment would be discontinued.

It is important to discuss these options with your doctor. In particular, a decision to consent to a trial of intervention without a definitive time limit needs to be based on a great deal of trust between you and your doctor. Let us imagine two patients with known chronic kidney disease, both of whom wish to describe in advance for their doctor the terms of the trial of intervention of dialysis they would want. One patient desires a maximum two-week trial of intervention of dialysis, if a terminal illness or persistent vegetative state is present, and stipulates that if progress toward ameliorating the disease is not evident at two weeks, the therapy would be discontinued. The other patient, given the same circumstances, desires a trial based on the presence of medical benefit, stipulating that if no progress is being made in treatment of the condition, the therapy would be discontinued (regardless of the timing). The latter option is more open-ended but allows for implementation based on the absence or presence of medical benefit, which may become medically evident well before a set time interval has elapsed.

It is important to remember that a doctor is not *required* to initiate or continue a therapy just because you have agreed to have that trial of therapy. As discussed in chapter 2, if your condition is such that use of the therapy would be without benefit, there is no obligation on the part of the doctor to use it or continue it. When a person selects a trial of intervention, that person is conveying his values and preferences regarding the use of that therapy more specifically than he or she would by simply agreeing to or refusing the treatment.

Why does the Values History ask me why I have made the decision I have made?

After your consent or refusal to each intervention, the Values History asks you why you have made this choice. This question gives you an opportunity to articulate the reasons, values, or experiences that influenced your decision. This information may be valuable to your doctor and family if such interventions are being considered when you are unable to speak for yourself.

In the next several pages we describe the various acute and chronic medical interventions included in the Directives Section of the Values History, in their order of presentation (the document itself appears in the Appendix). Reviewing what's involved in the use of these therapies will help you decide how you wish to respond to these items in the Values History. In addition to reading about these therapies here, you should discuss them with your doctor. It is important that you understand these therapies and the possible outcomes of their use before you complete the Values History (see chapter 8 for instructions on how to complete the document).

What is CPR?

Cardiopulmonary resuscitation, or CPR, refers to a broad spectrum of medical interventions that are employed to "restart" a person's heart or lungs after they have stopped working (that is, when they are said to be in a state of "arrest"). The methods used in CPR to attempt to restore bodily function include the manual compression of the chest, accomplished by pressing vigorously on the chest with both hands, and electrocardioversion (or electrical shocking of the chest), both of which are performed in an attempt to restart the heart, as well as introduction of air into the lungs by means of a mask over the mouth and nose or by means of an endotracheal tube (which allows oxygen to be delivered directly into the lungs). Cardiopulmonary resuscitation may also take the form of an injection of any of a vast array of cardiac medications that are used to attempt to restore normal electrical conduction within the heart after an arrest has occurred.

It should be noted that CPR efforts, performed with the intent of benefiting the patient, might carry unwanted or undesirable burdens. These efforts may result in rib fractures, electrical burns of the patient's chest, or a pneumothorax (the introduction of air between the lungs and the chest wall). An endotracheal tube may cause pain when introduced into the patient's respiratory system to control breathing during this emergency. CPR may be carried out with the intention of benefiting the patient, but there is potential for discomfort as a result of such efforts.

What is a ventilator?

A ventilator (also called a respirator) is a mechanical device that provides artificial respiration (breathing) by the person's lungs when the person is unable to breathe on his or her own. A ventilator controls the number of breaths the person takes each minute, the volume of the breaths, and the percentage of oxygen in each breath. A ventilator permits the doctor to maintain precise control over the breathing of the patient. A ventilator can be put in place either through a tracheostomy (the surgical insertion of a tube through the neck into the windpipe) or through an endotracheal tube.

What is an endotracheal tube?

An endotracheal tube is a clear plastic tube that is inserted into the mouth and down the throat by way of the vocal cords to the trachea. It allows for the free passage of air between the mouth and the lungs. The endotracheal tube is used to ensure that a patient's airway remains open when cardiopulmonary resuscitation is performed or a ventilator is used. (Long-term use of a ventilator usually requires the surgical procedure known as a tracheostomy.) The endotracheal tube is an intervention that many people, particularly people with chronic lung disease, have negative feelings about, based on past personal or family experiences.

What are nasogastric tubes, gastrostomy tubes, and other enteral feeding tubes, and how do they relate to nutrition and hydration?

A feeding tube delivers food to a person when the person is unable to eat by mouth or when it is not medically safe for the person to eat by mouth. The food is processed so that it is easily delivered to the person through the tube. Feeding tubes are medically indicated when there is a good chance that food delivered by mouth will be accidentally aspirated (diverted) into the lungs, resulting in aspiration pneumonia.

A nasogastric tube is a feeding tube that is placed through the nose, down the esophagus, and into the stomach. (The esophagus is the body's connection between the mouth and the stomach.) A gastrostomy tube is placed into the stomach or small intestine through a small hole surgically opened in the side of the abdomen. Such tubes may also be referred to, less specifically, as enteral feeding tubes, since they can also deliver food into the small intestine (*enteral* means *intestinal*). An enteral feeding tube is usually used when it is anticipated that the patient will not regain the ability to eat by mouth.

What is total parenteral nutrition?

Total parenteral nutrition, also known as TPN, is a method of providing nutritional substances by central intravenous infusion. For example, the intravenous solution may enter the right subclavian vein by a catheter in the right upper chest. TPN is generally used when a patient is unable to eat for a prolonged period and has difficulty digesting food. TPN is particularly beneficial for temporary use after an operation has been performed on the gastrointestinal tract. Because nutrition is provided straight into the bloodstream, entirely bypassing the stomach and bowels, these organs have a chance to rest and heal. When someone is unable to process food in the gastrointestinal tract for a longer duration, however, it may be necessary to use TPN for a sustained period of time.

What do intravenous medication and intravenous hydration mean?

Intravenous medication means having medicines administered into a vein; intravenous hydration means having solutions administered by vein to provide your body with necessary fluids and chemicals to sustain life. A directive concerning these two interventions would be appropriate in such diverse settings as hospital, home care, hospice, and long-term care.

Should you become terminally ill or enter a persistent vegetative state, medicines intended to treat your illness would not be administered intravenously if you state beforehand that you consider such treatment to be fruitless under those circumstances. On the other hand, medicines necessary for the control of pain *would* be administered, and other comfort care measures *would* be provided, should you become terminally ill or be in a persistent vegetative state. Similarly, life-sustaining fluids would not be administered if you state beforehand that receiving such fluids would not be acceptable to you if you were dying or if you were permanently unable to wake up.

What does "all medications used for the treatment of my illness" mean?

This language refines the intent of the directive about intravenous medication. It specifies consent to or refusal of *all* methods of medication delivery. With this directive you can accept or refuse oral medications, rectal suppository medications, transdermal (skin patch) medications, subcutaneous medications (injected under the skin), and injections of medications into the muscle, as well as intravenous medication, in the circumstances of terminal illness or persistent vegetative state. *With an all medication refusal directive, the use of pain medication to alleviate suffering would still be acceptable and permitted.*

What is dialysis?

Dialysis is a process whereby the blood is filtered through a machine that removes waste from the blood when the kidneys can no longer perform this function. Dialysis may be needed acutely—that is, temporarily—in response to acute kidney failure (such as kidney failure caused by infection or immune system disorders), or it may be performed indefinitely, if, for example, a chronic disease or other damage has caused a person's kidneys to fail without expectation of recovery.

What is an autopsy?

An autopsy is a procedure wherein a body is examined after death to find out what led to death. The reason for a person's death is often unclear, but by examining the body's organs, a medical team can usually determine what the cause of death was.

We recommend that you consent to an autopsy in an advance directive, because autopsy results are helpful. An autopsy provides the family with useful information, particularly if the disease that caused death is one that may afflict other family members. Autopsies help the medical team better understand the nature of the disease that caused death and may advance understanding of the disease. Thus, an investigation into the cause of your death may be helpful to others. Be assured that after autopsy, your body will be returned to your family for any desired religious services and burial that you or they request. Autopsy is not disfiguring to the portions of the body that would be visible if you or your family wished to have an open-casket service.

In some states, autopsies may not be carried out without the family's consent except when required by statute or court order. By clearly stating your wishes regarding autopsy in an advance directive, you may help your family decide to respect your wish for an autopsy and to provide the necessary consent.

What is organ donation?

Organ donation allows you to make a gift of your organs or other tissues (for example, your heart, liver, or corneas, or grafts from your skin) to others after you have been declared dead by your doctor. All fifty states have organ donation laws that allow you to specify the way in which you would like to help others through the use of your organs, whether by transplantation to a recipient, for scientific research, or for medical education. The magnanimous act of organ donation benefits other people either directly or indirectly.

Can my advance directive for organ donation be overridden?

The 1968 Uniform Anatomical Gift Act (on which most state donation laws are based) had no provision regarding family withdrawal of consent for an organ donation; the 1987 version of the law specifically states that a gift not revoked by the donor before his or her death is "irrevocable and does not require the consent or concurrence of any person after the donor's death." Nevertheless, health professionals *do* ask families whether they wish to allow organ donation, and family dissent does sometimes result in a valid gift being overridden. We believe that if an individual competently consents to organ donation, and if this consent is documented on an organ donor card, it would be morally wrong for the family to attempt to overrule such a directive, and it would also be morally wrong for the health professional to honor such a request from the family. The physician can and does play a mediating role in such cases, but the physician should honor the request of the patient and should withstand attempts by family members to override a valid organ donation. The physician's best response to such efforts is to educate the family about respecting the personal medical decisions made by the deceased relative and to highlight the intended altruism of the relative in donating organs after death.

What does it mean to be admitted to the intensive care unit?

When a person is admitted to an intensive care unit (or ICU) it means that the person is so severely ill that he or she requires intensive monitoring and intervention. Such monitoring may include the use of special catheters inside the large arteries or veins to monitor blood pressure, and the use of devices and medications to maintain blood pressure. The level of nursing attention is much greater in the ICU than on a medical floor of the hospital, because the ratio of nurses to patients is much higher.

There are many forms of medical interventions that can only be administered in the ICU. For example, in some hospitals, because of the many possible complications, certain drugs can be given only to patients being monitored in the ICU.

How can I decide what my preference is for an advance directive regarding ICU admission?

When you have already decided to refuse other medical therapies, you may wish to refuse to be admitted to the ICU. On the other hand, you are free to consent to ICU care for the increased attention received by patients there, while still refusing specific therapies that are used in the ICU (for example, certain drugs or the ventilator).

What does it mean to request that 911 not be called if I am at home or in a long-term care facility?

A person receiving care at home or in a nursing home (or in another long-term care setting) can direct the health care team not to take him or her to an emergency room and not to hospitalize him or her in the case of a sudden or worsening illness. This directive would allow the illness to run its natural course. There would be no attempt at emergency intervention by the paramedics or by health professionals at the emergency room or the hospital.

A person can refuse *admission* to a hospital but still request transportation to and *evaluation* in the emergency room. If this is your wish, you should write this directive out in your Values History. Such a directive requires that the administration of any therapy being considered not entail admission to the hospital. This means that, faced with a worsening illness, you do not want to be hospitalized, even if that is the only setting in which a specific therapy can be administered. This directive does not preclude the use of other medical therapies at home or in a hospice or long-term care facility, unless you have refused them as well, or unless they are not appropriate to your care. Also, many states have now passed laws to allow emergency personnel to provide comfort care without transport to the hospital, as long as you have signed a state-specific declaration to this effect.

What other advance directive options might I add to the Values History?

There are so many specific medical options that could be added that it may be best to agree that the agent appointed by your durable power of attorney for health care will make such decisions. But if you feel strongly about certain therapies not specifically identified, you can state your preference in the space provided in the Values History. You may feel strongly about certain surgical interventions or the use of certain life-prolonging medications, for example, or you may have preferences about nursing home placement or other environments of care.

You may want to request that a no-CPR order be enforced in the operating room if you are terminally ill or in a persistent vegetative state. Most surgeons and anesthesiologists prefer *not* to have a no-CPR order in the operating room; they prefer to be free to employ all possible means to return the patient to his or her preoperative state of health or better. You may or may not want to include this topic as a directive in your Values History.

What is proxy negation?

Proxy negation, a concept devised by Drs. Doukas and McCullough (not a standard legal term), allows you openly to name a person or persons whom you would *not* want to make decisions for you if you were unable to communicate. Such a decision is a weighty one. Your decision to name someone in this manner may arise out of your concern over conflict of interest or out of your perception that someone would request more or less treatment than you wish for your medical condition, as a result of personal conflicts, lack of communication, or differing philosophical or religious beliefs. We have found proxy negation to be appealing both to health care providers and to patients, because it attempts to exclude the voice of a designated person (such as Cousin Bob, mentioned previously) from consideration in a patient's care decisions, based on the patient's perception that this person will not act in accord with the patient's preferences, values, or best interest.

How will pain be treated if I'm terminally ill?

When a patient who has been diagnosed as having a terminal illness refuses life-prolonging treatment, pain control continues to be a medical concern. Even if a patient has refused other therapeutic interventions and medications, the patient is not considered to have refused pain medications. Since the intention of the doctor is to help the patient, allowing the patient to suffer pain is contrary to the doctor's goal of relieving suffering. Therefore, the doctor attempts to provide the best possible pain relief whenever pain is present during illness.

The side effects of pain medications can cause difficulties, however. Pain medicine can cause the level of the "breathing drive" in the brain to decrease, for example. Some people are concerned that the use of pain medications during terminal illness may cause the death of the patient by interrupting this breathing drive. We believe that one must look at the intent of the pain medication, and that is to alleviate pain, not to cause the death of the patient. If we imagine ourselves suffering from a terminal form of a painful illness, such as cancer, we can see that it would be a very rational decision to want that pain controlled by whatever means necessary, even if that level of pain control might result in death. The important distinction between giving a pain medicine that may have a lethal side effect and actively killing the patient is that the intent of the former is to benefit the patient by relieving pain, while the intent of the latter is primarily to end life.

All of these medical interventions in the Values History sound painful and intrusive. Why would I even want to consider them?

Any medical therapy has the potential of benefiting you as well as the potential of harming you. What you need to weigh are, first, the level of burden you are willing to accept in receiving a therapy and, second, how much benefit you would expect from that therapy. In all cases, we believe your doctor should work with you to help you understand these therapies and any other health care options, such as hospice care. Any pain you would experience should be treated with medication to alleviate your suffering.

How can I choose a therapy when I don't know what I'll be sick from?

Because people can't predict all the circumstances in which they may find themselves, many people think the best approach is to designate an agent or proxy, someone who can make a decision based upon the circumstances existing at the time the decision must be made, instead of giving specific advance instructions. But this is not always the best way to handle future uncertainty.

Although it is, of course, impossible to predict the future, many of us know the types of illnesses we are susceptible to, given our family tree, our past medical history, and our past and present habits. Given this information, it is wise, in our view, to provide guidance for one's proxy, family, and doctor by stating preferences for or against the use of individual medical interventions, as described in the Values History. Any of the interventions described in the Values History may be required for your care someday should you become terminally ill and incapacitated, irreversibly comatose, persistently vegetative, or in advanced dementia with incapacity. Again, conversation between you and your loved ones is essential to their understanding the context of your values and preferences for your future health care.

In each case there are consequences to your choices. Refusal of a particular therapy may mean that the underlying disease will end your life sooner, while requesting a therapy may entail prolonging the course of that disease and extending the duration of discomfort. Further, therapies can have uncomfortable consequences, such as the trauma to your system if your body is subjected to a cardiopulmonary resuscitation. These considerations must be balanced by the consideration of whether you feel your body could survive such a therapeutic attempt if you had a terminal disease or were persistently vegetative. Only you know what is tolerable to you in terms of pain, burden, benefit, and hope. It is best to discuss considerations such as these with your doctor, who can further inform you of the medical consequences of your decisions. Sharing your medical values with your doctor will help facilitate the decision-making process.

7

You, Your Family, and Health Care Decisions: Choosing a Proxy

Suppose you are ready to go ahead with an advance directive and are trying to decide who your proxy decision maker should be. What factors should you consider in choosing your health care agent, and what should you discuss with that person regarding your medical values and preferences for future treatment?

What guarantees that I get to make the final decisions in my advance directives?

The right to make choices about your own health care is protected *by law.* No one else is allowed to make those decisions for you—not your family, not your doctor—if you are able to make a decision or if you have already signed an advance directive or stated your concerns while competent. If, in addition, you have had a meaningful discourse with your loved ones on what you want in the future, you can feel even more confident that your wishes will be followed.

Decisions about health care are deeply personal, for they have many implications for your future. Making such decisions requires self-reflection on the values you hold dear.

What if my family doesn't approve of or accept my advance directives?

Your advance directive is a legal document made *by you, for you*. No one can overrule it if you were competent when you signed it (although some states limit the choices of advance directives available to you). Even if your family doesn't approve of an advance directive that you've signed, your word (through the directive) stands up against anyone's attempt to overrule it, including attempts by family members, such as Cousin Bob.

If the decisions are mine, why should I name a proxy?

Conflicts sometimes occur between family members about what a patient would want. That is why it is important to indicate not only what your treatment preferences are, but also who should speak for you if you are unable to speak for yourself. Your proxy can execute your choices despite family conflicts. Once you have decided who your proxy will be, you should discuss your preferences and values very carefully with him or her. You also should explain, briefly, to your family why you have chosen the person or persons named to represent you and describe in general what decisions you have asked them to make. It is a good idea to write some of this information down and give it to your agent. The written explanation will help your agent deal with family members or others who may not fully understand your wishes.

Explaining your preferences in advance helps people to accept them when the time comes. It also avoids misinterpretation of your preferences. For example, an ethical quandary often arises after a relative (recall Cousin Bob) arrives on the hospital scene to see the now ill and noncommunicative patient. The relative, who may not have communicated with the patient for a long time, then orders that "everything possible be done." Regardless of his or her love and devotion for the patient (and perhaps guilt over family issues that the medical team doesn't know about), this relative is making the waters murky, not clarifying them.

Your health care agent, if the two of you have discussed your values, beliefs, and preferences, will be able to make decisions based on *what you would want,* when you are unable to speak for yourself, to choose what you would have chosen had you been able to communicate your wishes. There is little benefit in naming a proxy to act on your behalf and then not discussing your medical values and health care preferences with that individual.

When considering using a proxy, the essential component is *communication.* Communication between patient and agent must be reliable and preferably ongoing, so that your proxy's understanding reflects your current thinking. It's best also to have frank and open conversations with the rest of the family now, so that there are no misconceptions concerning what you would want in the way of medical care. This prevents the values and beliefs of other family members from interfering with your wishes.

Why does interpersonal conflict occur?

Interpersonal conflict occurs when there is a difference of opinion or values between two persons, both of whom may believe they are acting in the patient's best interest. This can happen within the family when the patient has a specific set of values and beliefs that conflict with the values and beliefs of someone else within the family. It usually occurs when there is a difference of opinion regarding what constitutes overtreatment or undertreatment.

Sometimes a family member wishes to initiate treatment or continue to treat because the relative so deeply wants the patient to continue living that he or she either doesn't look closely at the preferences of the patient or believes that these stated preferences don't represent what the patient would really want now. Also, it is possible that a conflict of interest—due to ill will, or concern about cost or other burden of care, or a desire to receive an inheritance—may prompt a family member to undertreat an incapacitated person. In any of these instances, a family member might wish for the patient to be undertreated, regardless of the patient's desire for continued treatment.

As family physicians, we have encountered many family conflicts. These emotional interpersonal conflicts may be brought to a head when the family is burdened with the stress of a dying or persistently vegetative patient. Advance directives are very helpful in preventing or minimizing such conflicts, because decisions regarding your health care will already have been made—*by you.* Otherwise, your doctor will have to sort through the many emotions and agendas within your family to determine who might best speak for you. In our experience, this latter way of making these important decisions does a disservice to your family, your doctor, and, most importantly, you.

Whom can I appoint to speak for me?

You can transfer the right of making decisions to someone in your family or to a friend or loved one, as we have discussed before, by signing a durable power of attorney for health care. Several states allow living wills to include the naming of a proxy (you'll need to consult your own state's laws to determine whether your state permits this).

Your agent must not have any conflict of interest regarding the decisions he or she will have to make. He or she is responsible for conveying your values and preferences when you are no longer able to speak, and his or her values, beliefs, financial concerns, or other interests must not present a conflict of interest that could affect your care adversely.

Can a family member speak for a patient if the patient did not execute an advance directive?

In some states the family can do so. Several states have statutes that allow a family member to speak for the patient without a durable power of attorney for health care. Even in those states, however, if you want a *specific* person to make your health care decisions, you must name your agent or proxy explicitly through a durable power of attorney for health care.

In states without such laws, the family will be included in discussions about the patient's treatment, but the doctors may not be legally obligated to follow the family's instructions if the instructions lack clarity or specificity. If families do guide the patient's health care, they should aim to base decisions as much as possible on the general values and beliefs of the patient rather than on their own preferences. In this way, the family can actively apply the patient's belief system when the patient is unable to talk for himself or herself. Ultimately, this concept was of critical importance to the Nancy Cruzan case (discussed in chapter 8).

Sometimes family members don't agree about what a patient would want under current circumstances. To prevent conflicts, as we have stressed throughout this book, it is best to document your medical preferences now. People who have conversations with their families about their values and preferences (before and after signing an advance directive) can feel confident that their wishes will be carried out in the future. Through these conversations, family members gain an insight into each other, and this knowledge will make it easier for them to speak for each other if the need ever presents itself.

What is the family covenant?

The family covenant is a concept developed by Dr. Doukas. The family covenant document (see Appendix of this book) is an ongoing health care agreement that articulates how decisions are to be made within the family. The patient designates the doctor and those other family members, loved ones, and friends who will be within the family covenant. This agreement is an ongoing means of stating the following: *"These are the people I trust—and here is how I want them involved in my future health care."*

A family covenant is based on open communication and trust among willing persons closest to the patient. This agreement makes overt something that is commonly unspoken: *"Here is what I believe, here is what I want, and here is whom I trust."*

The physician would serve the role of facilitator in ongoing discussions in the patient-physician-family triad. With a family covenant, moral dilemmas can be transformed into meaningful moral discourse. The family covenant allows for a flexible agreement to bind those who choose to be entrusted with each other's interests. For advance care planning, it allows for families to set boundaries of what information can be exchanged with whom, how privacy can be expected to be honored, and how the proxy is to make decisions, such as how other family members are to help inform the proxy in making decisions. This model adds a family context to advance directive planning by designating not only the proxy but other relevant loved ones and how they can assist you when you cannot speak. The proxy then has a support network identified by you, with roles specified by you. The family covenant, then, is a model of how your family works and how you want it (and expect it) to protect your future interests when you cannot speak for yourself. It also allows you to select which doctor(s) and which family member(s) and friend(s) you consider trustworthy for inclusion. At the same time, the family covenant can identify individuals whom one does not want involved in future health decisions; this provision would benefit many families in which the members do not necessarily all see things the same way. Importantly, those not identified as part of the covenant (or explicitly excluded) would not be given credence as representing your values and preferences, and would only be treated as loved ones who do not have standing in your private health affairs. This model may help with your own potential Cousin Bobs.

What issues should I discuss with my proxy and family?

In addition to medical preferences, you may want to discuss your general values, your religious values, and your philosophical values. Having an understanding of your values will be very helpful to your proxy if you are unable to speak for yourself. These values are of particular importance when medical events don't occur as you had anticipated. A discussion of your values and preferences may include issues such as where you would like to live and how you would like to be cared for should you become frail or incapacitated. Choices concerning home health care, assisted living, and nursing home placement can be discussed. You may want to state your preferences among the alternatives that are available for nursing home care, specifying, for example, what kind of environment you would prefer. You may also address what form of religious or memorial service (if any) you would want performed after your death, and you may state your preferences regarding burial, cremation, or donation of your body. These topics should be discussed with your proxy, any alternate to your health proxy, and with any family or friends whom you want to help in these decisions.

What happens if I become unable to speak for myself and I haven't yet discussed my medical values and preferences?

Someone will have to make these decisions for you. If you have not discussed your values or preferences, and if you have not executed a written directive, members of your family (or someone else) will make decisions based on what they *think* would be in your best interest. Their judgment may not be the same as yours. By not signing an advance directive, you may burden not only your family (who will have to make painful decisions for you without the benefit of insight into your preferences) but also yourself, for you may be subjected to treatments that you don't want. Again, it is best to have discussions with your family, friends, and physicians as soon as possible.

Wouldn't these discussions be enough to let my family know what I'd want if I couldn't speak for myself?

Different family members may give conflicting opinions about your care, all of them believing that what they say reflects your wishes and is in your best interest. These opinions may be based on a misunderstanding of your past statements concerning your wishes or values about health care; they may be held out of a loving concern to keep you alive at all costs (regardless of your past wishes); or they may arise without any regard for your best interests—they may be the result of a direct conflict of interest. Interpersonal conflicts can occur between family members for any number of emotional, behavioral, and monetary reasons. Such conflicts can wreak havoc on the family's attempts to make decisions on behalf of a person who can no longer speak for him- or herself. That is why it is best to name (and document through a durable power of attorney for health care) one person whom you want to make the decisions (and an alternate). It is also why written preferences are critical in helping your proxy make the decisions he or she must make. Here the family covenant would provide direction for how your proxy and other loved ones could best serve your health care interests. If problems occur, assistance by your doctor is essential in facilitating renewed communication.

What if my doctor suspects a conflict of interest on the part of my proxy?

If the physician suspects a conflict of interest on the part of your proxy concerning what would be best for you, the physician can call on other members of the family in consultation to try to reach a consensus within the family, or, in most hospitals and some nursing homes, the physician can call on an ethics committee for advice on how best to treat you. Consultations by ethics committees allow for deliberations on medical cases that present a moral conflict. If this option is not available, the courts may become an arbiter in cases where conflicting medical viewpoints are heard; the legal ruling that results in these cases *must* be carried out.

What is a guardian or conservator?

A guardian or conservator is a person appointed by the court to take care of another person who has been deemed unable to make decisions for him- or herself. A guardian may be given authority to make all kinds of decisions (financial, health, and business), or the guardian's authority may be limited by the court to a specific area (the financial, for example). Depending on your state's laws, you may be allowed to specify whom you might want (or not want) to serve as your guardian in the future.

Do advance directives make it unnecessary for a guardian to be assigned?

Because advance directives, particularly durable powers of attorney, allow you to state your own decisions regarding health care, if you have such a document and a proxy, you won't need to have a guardian appointed to make health care decisions for you in the future. A durable power of attorney for health care also will be helpful to a judge who must decide whom to appoint if you need a guardian for non–health care matters. The durable power of attorney for health care, the living will, and the Values History—all can enhance medical decision making in case of your future incapacity, so that the need for a guardian for medical decisions might be eliminated.

8

SIGNING

ADVANCE DIRECTIVES

Suppose you are now considering signing an advance directive. Why should you sign now? What process should you use?

Why should I consider signing an advance directive now?

It's a fallacy to believe you can wait until you're approaching the end of your life to make advance directive decisions. Illness or accidents can happen *to anyone at any time.* Nancy Cruzan, for example, was only in her twenties when she had an accident that left her in a persistent vegetative state. (Her family's difficult situation is described in the pages that follow.) For this reason, we believe that adults need to make these advance directive decisions as soon as they can bring themselves to think about them. Otherwise, the family or the courts may be forced to make these decisions on their behalf in the future.

Why has the subject of advance directives recently received so much attention?

The attention of the nation was focused on this issue in 1990 by a landmark case decided by the Supreme Court. This case involved a young woman, Nancy Cruzan, who had been injured in an auto accident at the age of 26. The accident left her in a persistent vegetative state. The Cruzan family asked the U.S. Supreme Court to consider the case after the state supreme court in their home state of Missouri ruled against the family's wishes to withdraw the gastrostomy tube that had been providing life-sustaining nutrition and hydration to Nancy for six years. The Missouri Supreme Court ruled that Nancy Cruzan's oral wishes concerning medical care, which she had discussed with family and friends, did not constitute "clear and convincing evidence" of her intent. The U.S. Supreme Court upheld the right of the state of Missouri to require "clear and convincing" evidence, although they did not require that the evidence be in writing.

The U.S. Supreme Court's ruling in the Cruzan case gave great weight to the right of individuals to refuse life-sustaining medical therapy, including nutrition and hydration. Justice Sandra Day O'Connor's opinion focused attention on the fact that people do not take adequate advantage of opportunities to express themselves through a living will or durable power of attorney. For example, had Nancy Cruzan executed a durable power of attorney for health care, the family likely would have been able to carry out her stated wishes and discontinue use of the gastrostomy tube.

Several months after the Supreme Court ruling, new witnesses, previously unknown to the Cruzan family, came forward to offer corroborating testimony that Nancy Cruzan would not want to live on a feeding tube in a persistent vegetative state. With this testimony, which the trial court found to be "clear and convincing," Nancy Cruzan's preference—to discontinue therapy—was finally honored. Similarly, Terri Schiavo entered a persistent vegetative state after a cardiac arrest. After fifteen years of court and public fighting, Terri died after her feeding tube was withdrawn. This case, which occurred in Florida, was very different from Nancy Cruzan's in that the family was not unified in their support to withdraw treatment. Terri's husband and others had witnessed prior conversations regarding Terri's desire not to receive such treatments in the face of such circumstances. Terri Schiavo's parents, however, claimed that she was not in a persistent vegetative state, and they desired to continue her care. In the end, both the Florida Supreme Court and the U.S. Supreme Court (by declining repeated appeals) made clear that a proxy who has knowledge of witnessed preferences trumps the wishes of any other persons for an incapacitated person. Not surprisingly, advance directive requests have surged in the aftermath of Terri Schiavo's death. Maybe it is the Schiavo case that made you think that perhaps *now* is the time to fill out an advance directive.

Is age a factor in considering advance directives?

It seems natural that the younger and healthier the individual, the more likely he or she will postpone preparing an advance directive. Yet, many young adults have accidents that leave them permanently disabled. We ask the participants in our educational programs whether they have an advance directive, and usually a majority of them, whether they are young or old, health professionals or not, indicate that they have *not* prepared any type of directive.

Because of the Patient Self-Determination Act (discussed in chapter 1), young adults and older adults will be given information about an advance directive upon admittance to a hospital, nursing home, hospice, home health agency, or health maintenance organization. Therefore, we anticipate that more members of all age groups will begin thinking about these options.

We anticipate that the decisions in the Cruzan and Schiavo

cases will inspire many people, young *and* old, to attend to the preparation of an advance directive. That is our hope. There is no doubt in our minds that an advance directive provides clear and convincing evidence of a person's wishes.

In advance directive counseling and care, what differences can we expect according to age?

It is logical that middle-aged and elderly persons will be thinking more about the possible need for an advance directive and will have more frequent contact with the medical care system, through office visits to the doctor, hospitalizations, and nursing home admissions. The elderly may hear more about living wills and durable powers of attorney for health care in public education efforts directed to the "senior citizen" population, from presentations by state and local offices on aging, or within retirement communities. *All* adults are candidates for advance directives, however.

The young will confront the advance directive issue, too, though. On admittance to a health maintenance organization or whenever they are hospitalized for any reason, they will hear about this option for advance planning. Just as the elderly will be informed in many ways, and just as physicians will be kept up to date through educational sessions and review of procedural guidelines, the young will hear about advance directives, too.

We envision a process of cultural change in which young adults, for example, on an initial visit to a health maintenance organization for the purpose of giving a medical history and having a physical examination, will receive literature on the subject of advance directives and be asked to think about their values, beliefs, and choices so these ideas can be developed into an advance directive during a future set of visits. Although advance directives will more likely affect the lives of the chronically and acutely ill (and therefore mostly elderly people), we anticipate that advance directives will soon be understood as being beneficial for the entire society.

Are there different considerations for the young and old?

Many older persons seem to be more accepting of death than younger persons. They may demonstrate attitudes that reflect a sense of anticipatory readiness. Many chronically ill people wonder why they are still here, why they are still alive. People who are ill and are confined to hospitals or long-term care facilities, and people who are less active and have already given up much of their former independence, may demonstrate the greatest acceptance or readiness. Many older people are comforted by religious beliefs that help them look forward to their impending death.

In general, the elderly who are closest to death are more comfortable with the notion of death than those who are furthest from it; those who are furthest from death are less accepting and show greater denial and anger. The young man or woman who suddenly becomes terminally ill with a malignancy or AIDS will generally (and naturally) be in a much greater state of shock than the person in his or her eighties who has been chronically ill with congestive heart failure and emphysema and who has had repeated hospitalizations over the previous several years. The sixteenth-century French essayist Michel de Montaigne wrote that we could not endure sudden deterioration. "But," he wrote, "when we are led by Nature's hand down a gentle and virtually imperceptible slope, bit by bit, one step at a time, she rolls us into this wretched state and makes us familiar with it."

Do the issues that enter a person's Values History or advance directive change as a person ages?

It is certainly possible that one's choices in a living will or durable power of attorney for health care or Values History may change over time. As noted above, the younger person who is seriously ill may be in a state of shock, while the chronically ill elderly person who has been combating various health problems and declining over a period of years may be more accepting of death. They will both bring emotionally laden concerns to the process of wanting to complete an advance directive. Also, as we make the inevitable decline that goes with the passing of years, we may change how we feel about pain, control, and independence in our daily lives.

The ideal time for every adult to prepare advance directives, whether a living will, durable power of attorney for health care, or the Values History, is *when the individual is well*. It is best to sign advance directives after having taken time to reflect on the directives and having had discussions with family members and friends, your minister or spiritual advisor, your lawyer, and, particularly, your doctor. It's true that such a directive should be reevaluated periodically, in the same fashion that the will for one's financial estate should be reevaluated.

Why can't all this wait until later?

You never know when you suddenly will be unable to speak for yourself. Also, advance directives allow for decisions to be made on your behalf if you become incapacitated *temporarily* (for example, after an accident or surgery). By confronting the task of reflecting on your values and signing an advance directive now, you safeguard your right to control your health care in a way that no other present mechanism can. In this way, your ability to have therapies begun or discontinued will be facilitated if you are ever unable to speak for yourself. The vast majority of deaths occur in a hospital or nursing home, but when you are being admitted is not the time to reflect on your values and execute an advance directive. It is in your best interest to sign an advance directive *now*, rather than wait until you're admitted into a health care institution.

We must all appreciate that it is often hard to make such decisions when illness is not present and we are still fully competent. It is difficult to imagine the prospect of losing the ability to make our own medical decisions. We all demonstrate some denial, procrastination, and indecision. Understanding these human characteristics can make us feel less guilty, but we must nevertheless realize the importance of getting started and acting now.

Can't I just count on my family to decide?

That's a fairly heavy burden to place on someone else without the benefit of your input. You should exercise this responsibility directly, for your sake and for the sake of your family. Once you have made your own decisions, your proxy and relevant family members can then feel far more comfortable that they are making the best decisions on your behalf, all things considered. Advance directives free them of the need to guess what decision you would make. Also, as we saw in the Cruzan case, the courts may require clear and convincing evidence of your preferences, at least regarding termination of specific types of treatment.

Why do you think there is increased interest in active euthanasia and assisted suicide?

The subjects of active euthanasia (or mercy killing) and assisted suicide have become more visible in the public and professional literature and have captured the attention of the public. These subjects have been brought to the public's attention by the Kevorkian "death machine"; the assisted suicide "Quill" case in Rochester, New York; Oregon's state law permitting assisted suicide (recently unsuccessfully challenged by the Justice Department in the U.S. Supreme Court); Derek Humphrey's book *Final Exit;* and publicity surrounding the Dutch practice of legalizing euthanasia (when the patient *competently* requests it).

Almost everyone is concerned about the use of sophisticated technology on persons with advanced illness. Although modern treatments are often helpful, there is increasing concern from patients about the effort and the cost in physical, financial, and emotional terms during the last months of life when there is little benefit in such treatment. Many elderly people are angered by what they perceive as life-sustaining measures that are invasive, burdensome, and nonbeneficial, and therefore they are searching for other alternatives.

What's the difference between active euthanasia and passive euthanasia?

Much of the public discussion fails to distinguish between active euthanasia or so-called mercy killing, in which measures are taken that directly and actively cause the patient's death, and passive euthanasia, which refers to the withdrawal of treatments provided to the terminally ill or persistently vegetative patient. The public is done a great disservice when the terms *active euthanasia* and *passive euthanasia* are used interchangeably, either by the media or in doctor-patient discussions.

Active euthanasia can either be voluntary (the patient freely consents to actions that will cause his or her death) or involuntary (someone else, such as a family member or doctor, makes this decision). In either circumstance, active euthanasia represents a profound change in the doctor-patient relationship. The physician who participates in a mercy killing faces moral and legal issues very different from those faced by the physician who allows a patient to refuse treatments knowing that the refusal will result in death. In active euthanasia, the intent is to cause death, with immediate cessation of life resulting from a single act. In passive euthanasia, when the patient allows life-supporting measures to be withdrawn, the disease itself causes death.

Another distinction (discussed in chapter 6) is made between administering a drug to cause death and using a medication with the intention of alleviating pain and suffering even if the medication may have the additional effect of shortening life. Most people agree that the latter is far different from mercy killing or assisted suicide.

What alternatives exist to the practices of active euthanasia and assisted suicide?

What all people want as they confront life and death—and what we as physicians believe would arrest the demands for mercy killing and assisted suicide—are, first, alleviation of pain and suffering; second, avoidance of nonbeneficial and burdensome technological innovations that do not help the patient; and, third, a physician who will provide strength, support, and comfort. As physicians and as members of a larger community, we can provide the rational alternative to mercy killing and assisted suicide, by allowing patients the option of "dying well" (a phrase used in the literature by Dr. Arthur J. Dyck and Dr. William Reichel).

Physicians, nurses, and other health professionals involved in primary care medicine already provide comprehensive care, paying attention to the family and the home, and taking psychosocial issues into account. Your own primary care physician—whether a family physician or an internist—can help you to "die well." Helping a patient die well not only is a function of the physician's abilities to relieve pain and suffering but also relates to having respect for a dying patient's choices and wishes and values as expressed when ill and dying or as stated in an advance directive or by means of the patient's proxy.

The widespread use of advance directives may very well bring about revolutionary change. For example, many individuals now choose to die at home rather than in a hospital or nursing home as their illness reaches a point of finality. Supporting this decision is the success of the hospice movement, which emphasizes home care, as well as significant technological and pharmacological advances in palliative care, including improved knowledge and techniques for pain management in the home care setting. We can envision the hopelessly ill patient, young or old, choosing to remain at home in the advanced stages of illness, receiving care from family and friends, and having steadfast support and comfort provided by a physician, a nurse, and others.

Are there religious or spiritual considerations in the use of advance directives?

Considering the diversity of religious belief and experience in the United States, one can well imagine that some people may have a problem with advance directives, including living wills and durable powers of attorney for health care. Some may believe that any attempt to withhold a life-sustaining treatment, particularly nutrition, is wrong. Others may worry that living wills and other advance directives create a "slippery slope" that leads to active euthanasia and assisted suicide. However, most people believe strongly, as we do, that living wills and durable powers of attorney for health care—and, we would add the Values History—serve to promote individual freedom to stop nonbeneficial treatments rather than encourage active euthanasia and suicide. While rejecting practices that intentionally cause the cessation of life (active euthanasia and assisted suicide), the informed individual can at the same time reject burdensome, invasive, and nonbeneficial treatments by making certain decisions in advance. Discussing these decisions with your religious adviser may ease your mind; such a discussion allows you to reflect openly on the spiritual reasons for your choices.

We have met many elderly people who have strong religious beliefs affirming God or acknowledging the presence of a higher power or the Lord in their lives and who suffer health problems with dignity and serenity. These individuals have no problem stating their wishes and requests with great equanimity. They have lived a full life and, having accepted the possibility of death at any time, have written an advance directive.

The patient who affirms the presence of God in his or her life is empowered to make choices for palliative or comfort care and to make his or her wishes or choices known in advance. These choices may include rejecting life-sustaining treatments if the burdens of illness and the burdens of treatments cross a certain threshold.

Of course, there is a fine line between treatments that will benefit the patient and treatments that are burdensome and non-beneficial. Ideally, there is an ongoing, intimate dialogue between the individual and the doctor, so that each stage of the illness and treatment is evaluated and reevaluated. The patient may have survived many crises in which he or she benefited from medical therapy. With the illness advancing, the patient may feel that another round of invasive treatment for coronary artery disease, or another attempt at chemotherapy or radiation therapy for advanced malignancy, is simply beyond what he or she wants. At that point, the patient or his or her proxy designate may ask for comfort care measures, as in palliative care. Some or all medications may be discontinued, and an intravenous drip might be continued with morphine to reduce pain, such as in the case of advanced cancer, or to relieve severe congestive heart failure. The purpose of the morphine is not to end life but to keep the person comfortable.

In considering terminal illness, what is the role of hospice care?

Hospice care developed first in England (particularly at St. Christopher's Hospice under Dr. Cicely Saunders) and then spread to the United States, first to New Haven, Connecticut, in 1974, and then gradually throughout the country. The person accepted for hospice care is usually not expected to survive more than six months. The patient's physician is called upon to certify that the person likely will die within six months according to the natural course of the illness.

Hospice care is a philosophy of management of pain and suffering associated with dying. The palliative or comfort care manages the patient's pain, using pain medications in amounts necessary to guarantee that the patient is pain free. Clinical strategies or treatments that could prolong life are stopped. The hospice focuses also on the family or others who are providing care. It includes paying attention to the psychological, social, and spiritual aspects of care. In some circumstances hospice services are available around the clock, seven days per week.

Hospice care may be carried out at home, in hospice beds in hospitals and nursing homes, or in freestanding hospices. There are many variations of hospice care in the United States. Some hospices are part of home health agencies or work in tandem with a home health agency, providing special focus on hospice principles. The hospice provides case management and follows the patient as he or she might move back and forth between home and inpatient facilities. If necessary to improve control of pain and other symptoms, the hospice may place the dying person in an inpatient setting. If the caregivers at home simply cannot handle the dying person's needs, the hospice will place the dying person in a hospice setting at an inpatient facility.

Who are the members of the hospice team?

The patient's personal physician often does not play the key medical role in hospice care. Often a hospice physician takes charge medically. Alternatively, the patient's personal physician may work with the hospice team, backing up the nursing staff with telephone consultation and speaking with the patient and the family by telephone.

Every member of the team—physician, nurse, social worker,

and chaplain—is familiar with hospice principles. Hospice workers are highly skilled in methods of pain control and in working with terminally ill persons and their families. Hospice physicians and nurses have knowledge and skill in these areas that may not be found in the general medical and nursing community. We expect that in the future, education in medical schools, residency training programs, nursing schools, and continuing education programs will pay greater attention to hospice principles than has been paid to date.

Hospice has also created an army of trained volunteers who provide support for the patient and the family. A hospice volunteer's ability to enhance care, support, and comfort is remarkable. Many hospices also offer support groups for families facing the loss of their loved one. For more information about hospice care, or to locate a hospice in your area, write the National Hospice and Palliative Care Organization and National Hospice Foundation, at 1700 Diagonal Road, Suite 625, Arlington, Virginia 22314, or call 703-243-5900, or see their websites, at www.nhpco.org and www.nationalhospicefoundation.org.

Will my physician be willing to collaborate with me to develop an advance directive?

Because of the Cruzan decision and the Patient Self-Determination Act and most recently the tragic case of Terri Schiavo, physicians are more familiar with living wills, durable powers of attorney for health care, and other advance directives. Despite the findings of the national living will survey (discussed in chapter 5), things are changing, and many forces will work to involve the physician more actively in the preparation and use of advance directives. Expressing your wish to discuss advance directives greatly increases the chances that a conversation will take place between you and your doctor.

The physician is in the best position to discuss these matters, because he or she knows more about the person's health and illness, and what scenarios are possible, than anyone. The physician also understands the importance of the many relevant medical conditions: dementia, coma, persistent vegetative state, heart attack, ischemic heart disease and congestive heart disease, stroke, malignancy, and so on. The physician understands the use and implications of life-supporting therapies: ventilators, feeding tubes, dialysis, antibiotics, and cardiopulmonary resuscitation. Again, the discussion of an advance directive such as the Values History would best take place in the physician's office over a period of time.

There may be many forces working against the physician's active participation, however. Traditionally, for example, physicians have not spent time on advance directives but have concentrated on the treatment of illnesses or on preventive medicine, such as cholesterol reduction or Pap smears. The physician feels time pressures; increasingly, corporate and managed health care systems (such as health maintenance organizations and preferred provider organizations) are concerned with productivity. Also, physicians differ when it comes to values, attitudes, beliefs, and behaviors. For example, some are more interested in organic health, and others are more interested in a broader, "biopsychosocial model" of health. A physician may be preoccupied with treating the patient's chief complaint (for example, fatigue), and handling the patient's medical problems may consume all of his or her thoughts. Thinking and talking about possible future medical scenarios and advance directives may not occur to the busy, preoccupied physician.

Other demands placed on the physician may have prevented this task from rising to the top of the doctor's priorities. Some physicians, however, have systematically sent letters to their entire practice; in the letter the physicians offer a model living will, durable power of attorney for health care, or advance directive and invite the patient to come in to the office to discuss the matter. This is a very good sign.

Many physicians have received a copy of a patient's living will or durable power of attorney for health care and have simply placed it in the patient's chart for safekeeping without discussion. The physician should commend the patient for completing the document, thoroughly discuss the patient's decision and his or her understanding of it, and then file the directive. (On receiving and filing a directive, physicians should identify the file's contents by marking the outside of the patient's folder with a label that says: PATIENT'S LIVING WILL, DURABLE POWER OF ATTORNEY, OR ADVANCE DIRECTIVE IS FILED IN THIS CHART. The label also ought to state the date when the directive was received.)

While it is true that many physicians have not approached this new social trend with great energy or enthusiasm, few would openly reject a directive or express a negative philosophy on the matter. By discussing living wills, durable powers of attorney, and other advance directives with your physician, you will gain insight into your physician's attitudes, values, and behavior regarding the role of advance directives in his or her practice.

The future looks even brighter. Medical schools and residency training programs are now paying more attention to medical ethics—and particularly decision making around the end of life. Also, since passage of the Patient Self-Determination Act, physicians in practice are being offered workshops on end-of-life issues by the hospital medical staffs to which they belong and other sources, such as managed health care programs. Advance directives are turning up as a prominent topic in major medical journals and at continuing medical education courses. It is to be hoped that a long-term effect of the PSDA will be a wider acceptance of advance directives by physicians and their patients.

What if the physician objects to the action called for by the advance directive or the proxy?

A major difficulty that physicians may have with advance directives, living wills, or proxy decision makers is the potential for conflict between the dictates of the directive or proxy and the physician's opinion in a given case. For example, suppose the physician senses intuitively that this patient can be helped with surgery or another therapy. The physician may say that he or she wants to be governed by the patient's circumstances, not by a piece of paper. Some may say that patients cannot fully anticipate what their preference would be in a specific medical scenario, or that patients simply know too little about these matters to make decisions in advance. But these objections only add credence to the argument for physician training. The physician needs to learn how to educate the patient and how, through competent counseling, he or she can learn what the patient's values, attitudes, and choices are, as well as how to respect them. It is essential that people know that their wishes, not the wishes of a caring but paternalistic physician, will be implemented in the future.

Suppose the physician recently lost a patient who could have been saved had the physician not followed the patient's advance directives. Might that experience affect how closely the physician follows the next patient's advance directives? It shouldn't. Suppose a patient has become mentally incompetent since preparing an advance directive one year earlier, when he or she was fully competent. Might the physician say that, under the new circumstances, the previously stated wishes, choices, and directives are no longer valid? The physician shouldn't. Suppose the physician receives overwhelming pressure from the family to reverse the preferences of the patient, as stated in a competently written advance directive. Should the physician succumb to this pressure and overrule the patient's wishes? The physician shouldn't. Physicians are not to impose their desire to benefit the hopelessly ill patient with a specific treatment (under the guise of beneficence) and disregard advance directives that were clearly stated, just because the physician (or the family) believes that under the current circumstances the patient might have a different preference.

The well-known SUPPORT study revealed that physicians paid inadequate attention to end-of-life pain control and end-of-life preferences that were recorded while the patient was in the care of another health care provider. Physicians in this study did not write orders in the chart that reflected the patient's preferences, especially regarding when the patient wanted to refuse life-sustaining care. The study included an important intervention using nurse specialists, who served as advocates for patients and as a communication bridge joining patients, family, physicians, and hospital staff regarding efforts for symptom control. Two years of this intervention revealed that it failed to improve patient care or patient outcomes.

If a patient has a well thought-out advance directive to provide instruction to his or her proxy, these requests should be carried out. If the physician reviews this directive and finds aspects that are not reasonable, the time for dialogue between doctor and patient is early, when the patient is as well and competent as possible. Reviewing the advance directive and discussing it with the patient is an important contribution the physician can make.

The physician is bound ethically to follow the instructions of the advance directive or to transfer care of the patient to another doctor or health facility able to carry it out. It is best for both the patient and the physician to review the instructions of the directive soon after it has been written. This communication can clarify any ambiguity, as well as any reservations held by either party. The physician should also advise the patient to review the instructions with the designated proxy, and he or she can serve as a facilitator in discussions with the designated proxy and those family members and friends the patient selects. Advance care planning can be enhanced by engaging those who are closest to the patient, such as the family, so that they may participate in shared decision making according to the beliefs and preferences of the patient.

In the future, the necessary advance directive counseling skills should be built into the medical education and the continuing education of physicians, and reimbursement should be provided to the physicians who provide this counseling. Future standards of care should require review of these issues on a timely basis, just as the regularly performed Pap smear and cholesterol measurement are standards of good care.

What if my doctor doesn't condone advance directives?

Your physician has an ethical and, in most states, a legal obligation either to follow your advance directive or to make reasonable efforts to transfer your medical care to another doctor who will be able to follow the decisions, including refusal of treatment, that you've documented in your advance directive.

What if I change my mind about part of my advance directive?

As we have mentioned before, because this is a possibility, the advance directive should be reviewed periodically in the same fashion that a will providing for the disposition of a financial estate should be reviewed. While most people's choices are fairly stable from year to year, choices can change when our health changes, when relatives get ill or die, or even when famous medical ethics cases come under the media spotlight. We recommend that physicians make a point of reexamining advance directives with their patients on a regular basis. *You are free to change or revoke your previous treatment directives at any time.*

What is the best advance directive method?

Each vehicle has its own merits, and we do not favor one specific method over another. Living wills are designed primarily to provide for refusal of life-sustaining treatment should you become terminally ill, but several states allow their use for a person in a persistent vegetative state. The living will allows you to articulate directly (rather than through another person) your autonomous preferences, following specific instructions appended to the document (as allowed by most states).

A durable power of attorney for health care applies to any kind of medical decision that might need to be made if you are unable to communicate, whether or not you are terminally ill. It permits you to designate a decision maker and to specify the kinds of treatments you *do* want as well as those you *do not* want. Your agent or proxy can follow your instructions in the future. Together these documents provide even greater protection of your rights and interests.

The Values History is a powerful adjunct to either or both of these documents. It lets you identify your medical values and the specific medical treatments you would accept or refuse. It encourages you to *communicate* these preferences to your doctor, proxy, and family through a meaningful, reflective discussion.

Step by step, how should I document my wishes using the advance directives you've mentioned?

You can state your wishes about terminal illness through a living will and provide details about your medical values and advance directives through the Values History. These documents can be supplemented by the durable power of attorney for health care, which appoints an agent whose role is to make certain that your doctor implements your preferences. This approach focuses on treatment refusal in case of terminal illness. An alternative approach is to sign a durable power of attorney for health care and to supplement it with a Values History and a living will (for emphasis of those interventions you want and do not want in order to guide your agent).

If you work with an attorney to draw up a will or trust for estate purposes, the attorney may bring up the subject of advance directives. If he or she does not, you should ask your attorney about the various options of advance directives available in your state. If the attorney you are working with is not up to date on advance directives, our advice is to seek the help of a local attorney who is very familiar with advance directives in your state.

If you want to fill out your advance directives without an attorney, you have several options. First, you can obtain a living will or durable power of attorney for health care (usually for free) from a variety of sources: *You can download a free version of your own state's advance directives as listed in our Appendix;* you can also get copies of advance directives from your own family doctor, your local hospital administration office, your state attorney general's office, your health maintenance organization, your local state legislator, the citizen advocate group called National Hospice and Palliative Care Organization, or AARP (formerly the American Association of Retired Persons), as well as from other web links listed in our Appendix. After receiving a copy of the living will and durable power of attorney for health care, you should make photocopies of the blank forms for all adult members of your family.

Second, we recommend that you sit down with your doctor to discuss the meaning of signing these documents. You may want to make sure that plenty of time is scheduled for this component of your next medical visit when you make your appointment. Your doctor will be able to answer any questions you might have about the use or refusal of life-sustaining medical therapies. You should ask your doctor whether and when he or she would honor your right to refuse certain treatments.

You should make sure that the person you wish to speak for you agrees to serve as your agent in a durable power of attorney for health care. This is a role with the potential for significant responsibility, and the person ought to understand the significance of the role before agreeing to serve. It is also prudent to select an alternative proxy, who would serve if your first choice were unable to fulfill the task. Finally, after you have had these discussions and you have decided what your preferences are, you can fill out the forms. Sign the forms in the presence of two witnesses. *Be careful not to sign the advance directive until your two witnesses are present.* In some states, a notary public's acknowledgment of someone's signature can substitute for witnesses.

At this point you should make copies: one for your doctor's medical record, one for your agent, and one for each family member with whom you want to share this information. Extra copies should be made for good measure. If you are ever hospitalized, and the hospital (in keeping with the Patient Self-Determination Act) asks you if you have an advance directive, you can now answer yes, and you can ask a family member to bring a copy to be included in the hospital's medical record.

Considering the potential impact of these circumstances on your future brings up the issue of how a family covenant could be helpful to you. The family covenant is an ongoing health agreement among you, your doctor, and family members and friends whom you want involved in your future health. The agreement sets out, in your own words and terms, how you want information about you discussed with other covenant members, how you want decisions made if you can no longer make decisions, how you want your proxy to work with (or not work with) others in the covenant (and whom to exclude from decision making, if anyone), and how all those who freely enter this agreement should resolve their differences to avoid rancor (and courts). The family covenant more realistically acknowledges that your proxy will likely not be in a vacuum and may desire the support of loved ones whom you designate in making future decisions.

Such a conceptual framework can avoid family disagreements during health care crises and decrease the likelihood that family members or friends outside the covenant will attempt to undermine your values and preferences. This flexible framework is based on your forethought about how you see yourself within your family and the potential role these persons have in your future. It also can stipulate that some persons may be neither entrusted with your health information nor a party to future health care decisions. This concept is echoed in the Proxy Negation section of the Values History. Time and trust provide the ongoing nourishment of the family covenant. Trust is predicated on mutual care and conviction to respect the other parties of the covenant. So, what you put into this agreement is what you will get out of it.

Please also feel free to photocopy "**My Advance Directives for Future Medical Treatment**," found in the Appendix of this book. Use it to document what forms you have completed, including the family covenant agreement, and keep this form in a safe place in your home that is known to your proxy, family, and doctor. In case of a future emergency, medical personnel and your family and proxy will know which documents you have completed if you use this instrument to keep your health directives in order.

As a next step in the advance directive process, we recommend that you make a copy of the **Values History** found in the Appendix of this book. At this point, you may want to talk with your doctor, your spouse, and other family members about the values you consider important. The Values History is not intended to be a laundry list of things wanted and refused. The Values History is intended to be a springboard for reflection about what values regarding your future medical care you hold dear and how you would want medical decisions made based on these values. In turn, it is intended to spur reflection and discussion between you, your proxy, your other family members and friends, and your doctor. *This process makes autonomy a priority in what happens to you in your future, based on those things you value and have relayed to those you care about and trust.* These discussions need not, and should not, be rushed; you can discuss your values and preferences with your family, friends, or religious adviser over several months, and you can talk with your doctor over the course of several visits. This process will be most productive for you if it is reflective and introspective. You will know the best way—your own way—to complete this process. Remember that the Values History is intended to reflect your own values, not those of your loved ones, so do not feel compelled or swayed to do things that they would want for themselves, but base your preferences on your own medical values.

When you are ready, fill out the Values Section of the Values History, detailing those values that would be most important in your care if you were terminally ill and unable to communicate, were in an irreversible coma or persistent vegetative state, or were in end-stage dementia and unable to communicate. Also, explain why or in what way these philosophical, religious, pragmatic, or other values are important to you and your medical decision making. If you are presently ill, you may already have strong feelings in this regard. Discuss them at length with your proxy, family, and other loved ones. Write them down. This written record will let other people know about your medical values and how you wish them to influence your care in the future.

After you have completed the Values Section, continue to the Directives Section of the Values History. Before completing this section, review the medical interventions most relevant to your current medical condition with your family doctor. For instance, a person with known chronic lung disease may have very strong feelings about being placed on a ventilator, particularly if this person has been placed on a ventilator in the past. Also, reflect on what it means to be terminally ill and incapacitated, irreversibly comatose, persistently vegetative, or in advanced dementia with incapacity. By reviewing all of these treatment directives and ways they would be used in your future, you have a much better chance of accomplishing what a living will is intended to accomplish: completing an informed consent to request or refuse life-sustaining treatments.

In the Directives Section, you can specify which health care options you definitely would—or would not—select for yourself, by placing a check mark beside in the appropriate options. If you would like to specify a trial of intervention for specific health care options (as discussed in chapter 6), indicate that this is your preference; you can choose either a time-limited trial or a trial based on medically judged benefit. Remember that the option of a trial of intervention based on medically judged benefit requires a great deal of communication between you, your doctor, and your proxy to establish a clear understanding of your values and preferences. The space for other directives at the end of the Directives Section allows you to specify any additional medical therapeutic options whose use you wish to consent to or refuse.

If there are family members or other persons whom you want to disqualify from making decisions for you, those persons should be identified in the Proxy Negation section of the Values History. This directive informs your family, your agent on the durable power of attorney for health care, and your family doctor that this person is to have no standing regarding your care. This negation is similar to not including a family member in a family covenant for your future health care. The proxy negation is even more emphatic about excluding someone from being involved in your future health care.

You may also at this time wish to fill out an organ donor card, available from the department of motor vehicles in most states, so that if you die and your organs are still useful, you may give a gift of life or healing to another. Giving such a gift is a truly altruistic act.

Once you have completed the Values History (again, this may take some time and several office visits), we recommend that you photocopy the completed Values History and give a copy to your agent or agents, those individuals named in your durable power of attorney for health care. Along with your Values History, again, be sure to give your agent a copy of your living will and instructions (if any) in your durable power of attorney for health care, and make sure you discuss your preferences with your agent, family, and loved ones, to clarify your wishes. These documents and discussions will make it easier for someone to make decisions on your behalf if you ever are unable to speak for yourself, because your values and your treatment preferences will be clearly described therein. Any unforeseen medical circumstances will be much more easily resolved.

Very important: Give a copy of the completed Values History to your doctor.

Keep the original copy of your living will, durable power of attorney for health care, and Values History in a safe and accessible place in your home, so they will be quickly available should you become ill. *Do not put your advance directives in your safe deposit box,* because no one will be able to get them if you become incapacitated. Please also feel free to photocopy the enclosed **ADB Card (Advance Directive in Brief Card)** in the Appendix and use it to document which forms you have completed. Keep this card in your wallet, so that in case of a future emergency, medical personnel and your family and proxy will know where the copies of your document are kept.

You now have a very powerful set of documents to speak on your behalf should you ever be unable to make your own health care decisions or speak for yourself.

Why should I consider signing a living will when I could just sign a durable power of attorney for health care?

The durable power of attorney for health care is an important advance directive, but not everyone has a relative or friend whom they would feel comfortable appointing as a proxy decision maker. And not everyone has a surviving relative or close friend to consider for this role. The living will allows you to express your preferences and eliminates the need for a proxy decision maker. With a living will, even if you cannot choose a proxy (or if he or she is unavailable), you are still able to choose your own preferences for your future health care.

What should I do if there is no official living will statute in my state?

In those states without a living will statute (currently Massachusetts, Michigan, and New York), we recommend that you prepare these documents with the assistance of a local attorney who is well versed in your state's laws and legal rulings regarding advance directives. Advance directive forms for all states can be obtained via the web links listed in the Appendix. These forms might serve as a starting point for your own thoughts, your discussions with your family, and your formal discussions with your physician and attorney.

How should I think through my decisions?

It's probably best to think through the issues involved in advance directives over a period of weeks or months. It probably is not prudent to consider these important issues quickly, just to get something down on paper. We recommend that you reflect on these decisions with your loved ones and doctor before putting them down on paper.

Will I feel "settled" when I sign an advance directive?

In our experience, people who sign a living will or a durable power of attorney feel much more settled about the kinds of things that might happen should they be unable to speak for themselves. Having these preferences written down, and feeling confident that they will be respected, puts your mind at ease. Knowing that these decisions will not be left to other, uninformed, people and that your wishes will be followed even if you are unable to speak can be a great comfort.

Advance directives are an important part of future planning. They are best completed now, in the present, while you have the opportunity to voice your feelings about things that in the future you may not be able to share your feelings about.

In summary, it is best for people to sign advance directives when they are well and competent, and only after a discussion with their loved ones and personal physician. Ideally, the advance directive should be reviewed periodically, before serious illness occurs. The patient and family members whom the patient trusts should have time to have meaningful discussions on values and preferences in the advance directive and to share them with the physician. Advance care planning can best be enhanced by engaging those family members and friends who are closest to the patient, so that shared decision making will best represent the values and preferences of the patient in future health circumstances. This process is what we now hope you will do as you are **planning for uncertainty.**

APPENDIX

Links to Advance Directive Forms by State

The links below were collected by the authors from govern-mental, health system, and medical or law society websites as the most current at the time of publication of this second edition. The authors recommend using the state forms as a starting point in discussions with your physician and legal adviser and in making your own advance directive. In some cases, the living will form and durable power of attorney for health care (DPAHC) form are on different websites. These links are also accessible at the Johns Hopkins University Press website for this book at www.press.jhu.edu/books/title_pages/9306.html. A helpful alternative website for state forms, in case any of the links listed here prove to have been discontinued, is www.caringinfo.org/i4a/pages/index.cfm?pageid=3425.

Alabama
www.legislature.state.al.us/codeofalabama/1975/22-8A-4.htm

Alaska
www.hss.state.ak.us/pdf/advancedirective.pdf

Arizona
www.azag.gov/seniors/life_care/LifeCarePlanning.html

Arkansas
www.arkbar.com/whats_new/Advance%20Directive%20Information%20-%20for%20ABA.pdf

California
www.ag.ca.gov/consumers/pdf/AHCDS1.pdf

Colorado
www.thememorialhospital.com/tmhc.nsf/view/AdvancedDirectives

Connecticut

www.ct.gov/ag
(search for "Advance Directive")

Delaware

www.dhss.delaware.gov/dhss/dsaapd/advance.html

District of Columbia

www.dcha.org/Publications/AdvanceDirective.pdf

Florida

myfloridalegal.com/pages.nsf/Main/B18C541B29F7A7F88525
6FEF0044C13A

Georgia

Living Will: aging.dhr.georgia.gov/DHR-DAS/DHR-DAS_
Publications/LivingWill.pdf
DPAHC: aging.dhr.georgia.gov/DHR-DAS/DHR-DAS_
Publications/DPAHCVR.pdf

Hawaii

www.capitol.hawaii.gov/hrscurrent/Vol06_Ch0321-0344/
HRS0327E/HRS_0327E-0016.htm

Idaho

www2.state.id.us/ag/living_wills/LivingWill_DurablePower
OfAttorney.pdf

Illinois

www.idph.state.il.us/public/books/advin.htm

Indiana

www.caringinfo.org/files/public/indiana.pdf

Iowa

www.state.ia.us/elderaffairs/Documents/GiftofPeaceofMind
.pdf

Kansas

www.agingkansas.org/kdoa/publications/alzheimers/otr_
forms_nfo.htm

Kentucky

ag.ky.gov/livingwill/

Louisiana

Living Will: www.sec.state.la.us/pubs/Liv_Will_Dec_form
-1.pdf
DPHAC: www.ololrmc.com/workfiles/wills_durable.pdf

Maine

www.maine.gov/dhhs/beas/resource/adf.pdf

Maryland

www.oag.state.md.us/Healthpol/adirective.pdf

Massachusetts

www.massmed.org/AM/Template.cfm?Section=Search&
tem plate=/CM/HTMLDisplay.cfm&ContentID=10648

Michigan

www.michbar.org/elderlaw/pdfs/dpoa_hc.pdf

Minnesota

www.mnaging.org/advisor/directive.htm

Mississippi

www.msdh.state.ms.us/msdhsite/_static/resources/75.pdf

Missouri
www.ago.mo.gov/publications/lifechoices/lifechoices.htm

Montana
www.montana.edu/wwwpb/pubs/mt9202.html

Nebraska
www.hhs.state.ne.us/ags/advdir.htm

Nevada
dhcfp.state.nv.us/HIPAA/NV%20Law%20Concerning%20
Advanced%20Directives.pdf

New Hampshire
www.healthynh.com/downloads/endoflife.pdf

New Jersey
www.state.nj.us/health/ltc/advance_directives.pdf

New Mexico
www.phs.org/resources/documents/advance.pdf

New York
www.health.state.ny.us/nysdoh/hospital/english3.htm

North Carolina
www.ncmedsoc.org/pages/public_resources/death_and_
dying.html

North Dakota
www.legis.nd.gov/cencode/t23c065.pdf

Ohio
olrs.ohio.gov/ASP/olrs_AdvanceDirect.asp

Oklahoma
www.okbar.org/public/brochures/default.htm

Oregon
www.oregon.gov/DCBS/SHIBA/docs/advance_directive_form.pdf

Pennsylvania
www.aging.state.pa.us/aging/lib/aging/Advance_Directives_brochure1.pdf

Rhode Island
Living Will: www.rilin.state.ri.us/Statutes/TITLE23/23-4.11/23-4.11-3.HTM
DPAHC: www.rilin.state.ri.us/Statutes/TITLE23/23-4.10/23-4.10-2.HTM

South Carolina
www.scbar.org/pdf/public/LivingWill.pdf

South Dakota
Living Will: www.rcrh.org/Services/Patient/Docs/LivingWill.PDF
DPAHC: www.rcrh.org/Services/Patient/Docs/HealthCarePowerofAttorney.pdf

Tennessee
www2.state.tn.us/health/Boards/AdvanceDirectives/

Texas
www.texashealth.org/main.asp-level-2-id-DD579008B2CC42419E907944C83DBFE9

Utah
uuhsc.utah.edu/ethics/UtahLaw.htm

Vermont

www.vtpa.org/Advance%20Directive.htm

Virginia

www.vda.virginia.gov/pdfdocs/AdvMedDir.pdf

Washington

www.wsma.org/patients/who_decide.html

West Virginia

www.wvbar.org/barinfo/lawyer/will2.htm

Wisconsin

dhfs.wisconsin.gov/forms/AdvDirectives/ADFormsPOA.htm

Wyoming

www.caringinfo.org/files/public/Wyoming.pdf

Other Useful Links

U.S. Living Will Registry
www.uslivingwillregistry.com/forms.shtm

Caring Connections
www.caringinfo.org/

AARP
www.aarp.org/money/financial_planning/a2002-08-12-Estate
PlanningAdvanceMedicalDecisions.html

Department of Veterans Affairs
www.hsrd.research.va.gov/publications/internal/ylyc.htm

My Advance Directives for Future Medical Treatment

My name _____

I currently have signed:

[   ] Living will

Date signed _____

Where original kept _____

_____

Discussed with and copy given to:

[   ] My doctor

Name _____ Date _____

[   ] My proxy/health surrogate

Name _____ Date _____

[   ] Family members and other loved ones

Name _____ Date _____

Name _____ Date _____

Name _____ Date _____

Name _____ Date _____

Name _____ Date _____

[   ] Durable power of attorney for health care

Proxy name _____

Address _____

_____ Phone _____

Date signed _____

Where original kept _____

_____

Discussed with and copy given to:

[   ] My doctor

Name _____ Date _____

[   ] My proxy/health surrogate

Name _____ Date _____

[ ] Family members and other loved ones

Name _____ Date _____

Name _____ Date _____

Name _____ Date _____

Name _____ Date _____

Name _____ Date _____

[ ] Organ donation card

Date signed _____

Where original kept _____

Discussed with:

  [ ] My doctor

Name _____ Date _____

  [ ] My proxy/health surrogate

Name _____ Date _____

  [ ] Family members and other loved ones

Name _____ Date _____

Name _____ Date _____

Name _____ Date _____

Name _____ Date _____

Name _____ Date _____

[ ] **My family covenant:** I have entered a family covenant with my doctor, _____, and the following family members and friends: _____

_____

_____

_____

_____

If other family members or friends are not included above, they are not to be consulted about my health, given medical information without my consent or that of my proxy, and they are not to be part of any medical decision making on my behalf.

My family covenant directs members to carry out my autonomous values and preferences in the following way, in conjunction with my living will and/or durable power of attorney for health care:

[Potential areas for consideration:]
[   ] Who has access to my health care information (confidentiality)
[   ] Who else may participate in my health care decisions
[   ] Who is my proxy and whom else should he or she consult (or not)

_____

_____

_____

_____

_____

_____

_____

_____

_____

_____

_____

_____

_____

_____

_____

_____

_____

_____

_____

_____

_____

_____

_____

_____

_____

_____

_____

_____

_____

Signature _____ Date _____

Witness name/address:

_____

_____

Witness signature _____ Date _____

Witness name/address:

_____

_____

Witness signature _____ Date _____

This agreement has been discussed with and agreed to by the following persons, and a copy given to each:

[   ] My doctor

Name _____ Date _____

[   ] My proxy/health surrogate

Name _____ Date _____

[   ] Family members and other loved ones

Name _____ Date _____

Name _____ Date _____

Name _____ Date _____

Name _____ Date _____

Name _____ Date _____

The Values History

This Values History records my specific value-based directives for various medical interventions. It is to be used in health care circumstances when I may be unable to voice my preferences. These directives shall be made a part of my medical record and shall be used as supplements to my living will and/or durable power of attorney for health care if I am terminally ill and unable to communicate, if I am in an irreversible coma or persistent vegetative state, or if I am in end-stage dementia and unable to communicate.

I. Values Section

There are several values important in decisions about end-of-life treatment and care. This section of the Values History invites you to identify your most important values.

A. Basic Life Values

Perhaps the most basic values in this context concern length of life versus quality of life. Which of the following two statements most accurately reflects your feelings and wishes? Write your initials and the date next to the number you choose (initials/date).

_____ 1. I want to live as long as possible, regardless of the quality of life that I experience.
_____ 2. I want to preserve a good quality of life, even if this means that I may not live as long.

B. Quality-of-Life Values

There are many values that help us to define for ourselves the quality of life that we want to live. The following values appear to be those

*most frequently used to define quality of life. Review this list and circle
the values that are most important to your definition of quality of life.
Feel free to elaborate on any of the items in the list, and to add to the
list any other values that are important to you.*

1. I want to maintain my capacity to think clearly.
2. I want to feel safe and secure.
3. I want to avoid unnecessary pain and suffering.
4. I want to be treated with respect.
5. I want to be treated with dignity when I can no longer speak for myself.
6. I do not want to be an unnecessary burden on my family.
7. I want to be able to make my own decisions.
8. I want to experience a comfortable dying process.
9. I want to be with my loved ones before I die.
10. I want to leave good memories of me for my loved ones.
11. I want to be treated in accord with my religious beliefs and traditions.
12. I want respect shown for my body after I die.
13. I want to help others by making a contribution to medical education and research.
14. Other values or clarification of values above:

II. Directives Section

*The following directives are intended to clarify what you want and do
not want if one day you are terminally ill and unable to communicate, are in an irreversible coma or persistent vegetative state, or are in
end-stage dementia and unable to communicate. Some directives
involve a simple yes or no decision. Others provide for the choice of a
trial of a therapeutic intervention to determine medical benefit. Write
your initials and the date next to the number for each directive you
complete (initials/date).*

_____ 1. I want to undergo cardiopulmonary resuscitation.

    _____ YES

    _____ NO

    Why?

_____ 2. I want to be placed on a ventilator.

    _____ YES

    _____ TRIAL for the TIME PERIOD OF _____

    _____ TRIAL to determine effectiveness using reasonable medical judgment

    _____ NO

    Why?

_____3. I want to have an endotracheal tube used in order to perform items 1 and 2.

    _____ YES

    _____ TRIAL for the TIME PERIOD OF _____

    _____ TRIAL to determine effectiveness using reasonable medical judgment

    _____ NO

    Why?

_____ 4. I want to have total parenteral nutrition administered for my nutrition.

    _____ YES

    _____ TRIAL for the TIME PERIOD OF _____

    _____ TRIAL to determine effectiveness using reasonable medical judgment

    _____ NO

    Why?

_____ 5. I want to have intravenous medication and hydration administered. Regardless of my decision, I understand that intravenous hydration, to alleviate discomfort, or pain medication will not be withheld from me if I so request them.

_____ YES

_____ TRIAL for the TIME PERIOD OF _____

_____ TRIAL to determine effectiveness using reasonable medical judgment

_____ NO

Why?

_____ 6. I want to have all medications used for the treatment of my illness continued. Regardless of my decision, I understand that pain medication will continue to be administered, including narcotic medications.

_____ YES

_____ TRIAL for the TIME PERIOD OF _____

_____ TRIAL to determine effectiveness using reasonable medical judgment

_____ NO

Why?

_____ 7. I want to have nasogastric, gastrostomy, or other enteral feeding tubes introduced and administered for my nutrition.

_____ YES

_____ TRIAL for the TIME PERIOD OF _____

_____ TRIAL to determine effectiveness using reasonable medical judgment

_____ NO

Why?

_____ 8. I want to be placed on a dialysis machine.

_____ YES

_____ TRIAL for the TIME PERIOD OF _____

_____ TRIAL to determine effectiveness using reasonable medical judgment

_____ NO

Why?

_____ 9. I want to have an autopsy done to determine the
cause(s) of my death.

_____ YES

_____ NO

Why?

_____ 10. I want to be admitted to the intensive care unit (ICU).

_____ YES

_____ NO

Why?

_____ 11. If I am a patient in a long-term care facility or receiving
care at home and experience a life-threatening change
in health status, I want 911 called in case of a medical
emergency.

_____ YES

_____ NO

Why?

_____ 12. Other Directives

_____

_____

_____

_____ 13. Proxy Negation: I request that the following person(s) NOT be allowed to make decisions on my behalf in the event of my disability or incapacity:

_____

_____

_____

_____

I consent to these directives after receiving honest disclosure of their implications, risks, and benefits from my physician, being free of constraints, and being of sound mind.

Signature: _____ Date: _____

Witness name/address: _____

Witness name/address: _____

Adapted from David Doukas and Laurence McCullough, "The Values History: The Evaluation of the Patient's Values and Advance Directives," *Journal of Family Practice* 32 (February 1991): 145-53. Reprinted by permission of Appleton and Lange, Inc.

ADB Card

Advance Directive in Brief: To be used in my future care if I am terminally ill and incapacitated or if I am unable to consent in urgent circumstances.

Patient's name: _____

I currently have signed:

[ ] Living Will
Date signed: _____
Location: _____

[ ] Durable Power of Attorney for Health Care
Proxy Name: _____
Telephone: _____
Date signed: _____
Location: _____

[ ] Organ Donation Card
Date signed: _____
Location: _____

Signature: _____ Date: _____

Photocopy this card and place it in your wallet when completed.

Index